CAROTID ARTERY - GENDER AND HEALTH

Edited by **Rita Rezzani**
and **Luigi Fabrizio Rodella**

Carotid Artery - Gender and Health

http://dx.doi.org/10.5772/intechopen.73939
Edited by Rita Rezzani and Luigi Fabrizio Rodella

Contributors

Azran Azhim, A Rahman Rasyada, Jurek Olszewski, Piotr Niewiadomski, Mohamed Khaled Elewa, Renato Casana, Chiara Malloggi, Valerio Stefano Tolva, Andrea Odero Jr, Vincenzo Silani, Gianfranco Parati, Richard Bulbulia, Alison Halliday, Lachezar Manchev, Eduardo Waihrich, Bruno Parente, Paulo Gonçalves, Camila Damasceno, Elias Rabahi, Carlo Ontiveros, Fabio Fernades, Rosa Vona, Elisabetta Straface, Lucrezia Gambardella

First published in London, United Kingdom, 2019 by IntechOpen
IntechOpen is the global imprint of INTECHOPEN LIMITED, registered in England and Wales, registration number: 11086078, The Shard, 25th floor, 32 London Bridge Street
London, SE19SG – United Kingdom
Printed in Croatia

British Library Cataloguing-in-Publication Data
A catalogue record for this book is available from the British Library

Additional hard and PDF copies can be obtained from orders@intechopen.com

Carotid Artery - Gender and Health, Edited by Rita Rezzani and Luigi Fabrizio Rodella
p. cm.
Print ISBN 978-1-78984-981-3
Online ISBN 978-1-83962-189-5
eBook (PDF) ISBN 978-1-83962-190-1

For EU product safety concerns:
IN TECH d.o.o., Prolaz Marije Krucifikse Kozulić 3, 51000 Rijeka, Croatia,
info@intechopen.com or visit our website at intechopen.com.

Meet the editors

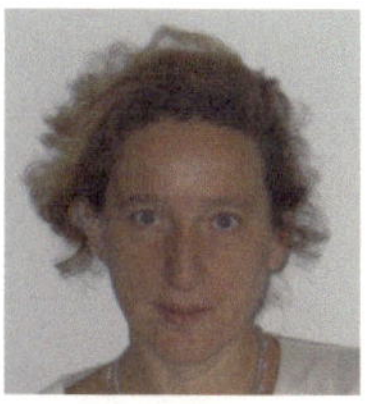

Dr. Rita Rezzani is Full Professor of Human Anatomy and Chairman of the Anatomy and Physiopathology Division of the Department of Clinical and Experimental Sciences, University of Brescia, Italy. She is also director of the Interdepartmental Research Center for the Study of the Adaptation and Regeneration of Tissues and Organs (ARTO) and author of more than 200 full-length publications focusing mainly on oxidative stress, cardiovascular diseases, aging and natural antioxidants. She is the author of books, book chapters and monographs on systematic anatomy, microscopic anatomy and ageing-related diseases and antioxidants effects.

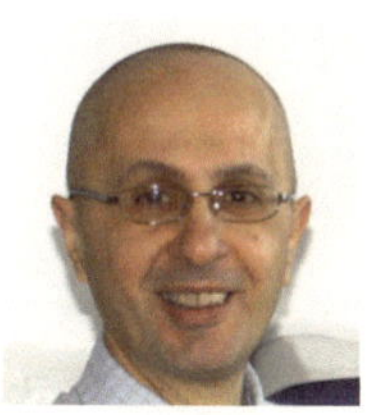

Dr. Luigi F. Rodella is Full Professor of Human Anatomy and Head of the Gross Anatomy Centre of the Anatomy and Physiopathology Division of the Department of Clinical and Experimental Sciences, University of Brescia, Italy. He is Deputy Director of the Interdepartmental Research Center for the Study of the Adaptation and Regeneration of Tissues and Organs (ARTO) and author of more than 200 full-length publications focusing mainly on craniofacial anatomy, cardiovascular diseases, tissue regeneration and pain transmission. He is the author of books, book chapters and monographs on systematic anatomy, microscopic anatomy, surgical anatomy and neuroscience.

Contents

Preface

Gender influences are an individual's way of living, becoming unwell, and seeking and receiving care. The failure to take gender into account in evaluating the pathway of health and disease, as well as in developing health policies and programmes, contributes to one of the many sources of health inequities.

There are many data reporting the different structures and compliances in vascular vessels and, in particular, regarding the carotid artery. Given the role of arterial wall elasticity in the development of cardiovascular diseases, carotid artery variations, compliance and its distensibility have been used as predictors of cardiovascular risk, although gender differences are a good point of scientific debate. Sex hormones play an important role in vasomotion and vascular remodelling, as well as vascular functions, and have been shown to change throughout the menstrual cycle. Estradiol has been shown to promote nitric oxide-mediated vasodilatation, reduce oxidative stress and retard atherosclerosis.

This book highlights the biological differences among women and men focusing on the updates of gender influence in carotid artery compliance in health and pathological states.

Prof. Rita Rezzani and Prof. Luigi Fabrizio Rodella
Anatomy and Physiopathology Division
University of Brescia, Italy

Chapter 1

Anatomical Anomalies of Carotid-Vertebral Arteries in Patients with Dizziness and Impaired Hearing

Jurek Olszewski and Piotr Niewiadomski

Additional information is available at the end of the chapter

http://dx.doi.org/10.5772/intechopen.78621

Abstract

Currently, Doppler ultrasound examinations are of particular importance, including continuous wave Doppler and color-coded pulsed wave Doppler. Excellent images are obtained using contrast computed tomography angiography (CTA) and magnetic resonance angiography (MRA), which give greater understanding of blood flow in the cranial and intracranial vessels under normal conditions and in pathological situations caused by both anatomical anomalies and acquired abnormalities. Our previous studies, concerning the analysis of the frequency and types of anatomical anomalies of the cranial arteries, i.e. vertebral and carotid arteries, in patients with dizziness and impaired hearing, demonstrated that hypoplasia of the right vertebral artery was the most common anatomical anomaly occurring in 58.7% of cases, of which 51.7% were women and 6.9% men; hypoplasia of the left vertebral artery, occurring in 24.7% of the study group, of which 13.8% were women and 10.3% men; hypoplasia of the right internal carotid artery found in 3.4% of women and of the left internal carotid artery in 6.8% of cases, 3.4% in women and 3.4% in men; and hypoplasia of the right common carotid artery was reported in 3.4% of men, whereas critical stenosis of the left subclavian artery with subclavian steal syndrome was observed in 3.4% of women. Although tinnitus was the most frequent symptom occurring in those patients, in this study dizziness was most common in patients admitted to the Department for the diagnosis, possibly because they found it more disturbing.

Keywords: anomaly, carotid, vertebral arteries, dizziness, impaired hearing

1. Introduction

The complex anatomy of cranial and intracranial arteries and the formation of collateral circulation have been studied for many years. Currently, Doppler ultrasound examinations are of particular importance, including continuous wave Doppler and color-coded pulsed wave Doppler. Excellent images are obtained using contrast computed tomography angiography (CTA) and magnetic resonance angiography (MRA) [1–3], which give greater understanding of blood flow in the cranial and intracranial vessels under normal conditions and in pathological situations caused by both anatomical anomalies and acquired abnormalities [4–8].

Anomalies of the vertebral arteries include: underdevelopment of one vertebral artery, coexisting with compensatory dilatation of the contralateral artery, total absence of one of the vertebral arteries, variations in vertebral artery origin from the aorta or from the common carotid artery, double origin of one vertebral artery forming a common vascular trunk, and duplication of the vertebral artery on one side [9].

The reduction of blood flow caused by a hemodynamically significant factor triggers numerous compensatory mechanisms. These include local regulation of the cerebral circulation, increase in systemic blood pressure and, in the case of permanent reduction of blood supply, the formation of collateral circulation [1].

Anatomical anomalies do not produce specific symptoms that could suggest early diagnostic tests aiming at their identification, and they often coexist with other disorders that can cause similar symptoms in the ENT organs (post-traumatic or degenerative changes in the cervical spine, hypertension, hormonal or metabolic disorders). Therefore, many authors are inclined to the view that in adults, anatomical anomalies are diagnosed only when other factors that impair the vascularization of the central nervous system are present in these patients. A possible example of this involves reports that indicate that hypoplasia of the vertebral artery is more common in menopausal women, who often suffer from symptoms of vertebrobasilar insufficiency [5, 6].

1.1. Anatomical anomalies of the intracranial vessels

The sense of balance and spatial orientation is conditioned by efficient functioning of individual elements of the system of balance and proper communication between them. Proper blood supply to each of its elements is one of the basic and necessary conditions of efficient functioning of this system [10–12].

It originates from intracranial vessels that, among other things, include vertebral arteries, merging and creating the vertebrobasilar system that supplies blood to a part of the brain, the inner ear, pons, cerebellum, and spinal cord. For proper functioning of the peripheral organ of balance, the most important is the labyrinthine artery that, in accordance with the declining frequency of anatomical variations, branches off from the anterior inferior cerebellar artery, basilar artery or vertebral artery and then, usually already in the inner auditory canal, divides into three branches: the vestibular artery, the vestibular-cochlear artery and the cochlear artery. Regardless of the anatomical variation, blood supply to the inner ear directly or indirectly arises from the vertebral artery identical on each side of the body.

The vertebral artery branches off from the ipsilateral subclavian artery with four possible anatomical varieties, with a prevalence of 0.1–90%, and for the branch-off from the vessel in relation to the thyroid-cervical trunk [13]. Its further course is divided into four segments:

- V1 – arises from the subclavian artery and enters the transverse foramen of C6,
- V2 – a segment of the vessel running from the transverse foramen of C6 to the transverse foramen of C2,
- V3 – a suboccipital segment, emerges from the transverse process of C2 to pierce the dura at the height of the *foramen magnum*,
- V4 – an intracranial segment, from the *foramen magnum* joins its contralateral counterpart at the lower border of the pons to form the basilar artery of the brain.

Some authors also distinguish the V0 segment, which is the site of branching off the vessel [16]. After branching off from the subclavian artery, the vertebral artery is directed upwards and enters the canal formed by the transverse processes of the cervical vertebrae, in 90% of cases at the C6 level, although possible are also entry variants at the level of the C5 (in 5%), C4 (2%), C7 (2%), C3 (1%). In the case of entry other than the C6 level, the vessel runs ventrally in relation to the transverse processes of the vertebrae located below, between the pre-vertebral muscles and the bone forming the spinal process. Next, it runs upwards vertically, surrounded by the spinal venous plexus and closed in the periosteal envelope derived from the periosteum of the transverse processes of the vertebrae, which forms two fibrous rings: proximal, in the place of entry to the channel, and distal, at the site where the vessel penetrate the dura mater. The fibrous rings are the only sites to integrate the vessel with the surroundings. The vertical course of the vessel changes above the height of the C3. This is due to the different construction of the spinal process of the C2 which, in contrast to the others, is set diagonally down in relation to the vertebral body, and, in addition, it is longer than the others. This makes the vertebral artery take the lateral and almost horizontal directions to reach the C2 transverse hole. Then it returns to its vertical course in a short section, from the C2 to the C1, to take its near-horizontal direction again, running in the sulcus of the C1 rear arch, and then it heads obliquely, vertically and medially, pierces the dura mater to continue in the intracranial segment. On the surface of the occipital bone, both vertebral arteries merge to form the basilar artery. The entire length of the artery is accompanied by the spinal nerve from the stellate ganglion which, together with the branches of the middle and upper cervical ganglia and branches of the cervical spinal nerves, forms the spinal plexus.

The spinal arteries in their course give off:

- muscular branches,
- spinal branches,
- meningeal branch,
- anterior spinal artery,
- posterior spinal artery,
- posterior inferior cerebellar artery.

Muscular branches seem to be particularly noteworthy. In addition to supplying the structures corresponding to the name of the branch with blood, like other branches of the vertebral arteries, muscular branches have connections with the relevant branches of the ascending muscular carotid artery, deep carotid artery and external carotid artery. Due to these connections, a vascular network is formed, that in the event of the closure of the proximal segment of the vertebral artery could allow it to refill with blood above the site of closure or narrowing and thus ensuring the proper functioning of the vertebrobasilar system. The vascular networks mentioned above do not need to be visible in the standard angiographic studies, which does not preclude their existence. Visualization of these anastomoses may require the use of special imaging techniques.

Basing on the data obtained at the Department of Otolaryngology, Laryngological Oncology, Audiology and Phoniatrics at the Medical University of Lodz, Poland, collected in the years 2007–2012 and comprising 2167 patients diagnosed as having dizziness and hearing disorders, anomalies of intracranial vessels were confirmed in 29 patients (1.3%) [9]. It could be expected that the incidence of such anomalies is greater than that shown above, as indicated by other authors who estimated the incidence of anomalies of the vertebral arteries in the population at a level of 31% in the case of isolated changes and 15% of the population in the case of two-sided changes, or a few changes within one vessel in its different segments [14]. The anomalies more frequently concern the left vertebral artery and can be isolated and coexist with other vascular anomalies related to the aortic arch or subclavian artery [4, 15]. **Figure 1** shows an example of complex anomalies.

The overview of the anomalies should start from the most prevalent ones, and such is the degree of asymmetry of their diameter, though it is generally considered an anatomical variant.

Differences in the diameter of these vessels range from small, virtually imperceptible in imaging studies, to substantial hypoplasia of one of the arteries with proper or increased width of the artery on the opposite side (**Figure 2**). Depending on the source, it is said that vertebral arteries vary in diameter in 40–75% of the population [6, 10, 11]. The study results unanimously indicate a higher incidence of domination in terms of the width of the left vertebral artery (50–65%), whereas the right spinal artery is wider only in 10–25% of the study population [11, 12]. The limit value of the diameter of the vertebral artery above which it is no longer asymmetry but hypoplasia is not explicitly specified. As a criterion for hypoplasia the diameter of the vessel amounts to ≤2 mm along its entire length [13], though some authors give a limit value of ≤3 mm, possibly extending the criteria for diagnosis of, disclosed in the ultrasound with Doppler, high resistance and reduced blood flow [14]. Other criteria are also used for eligibility of the vertebral arteries as hypoplastic, these are the degree of asymmetry between the vessels that, depending on the author, fluctuates between 1:1.7 [15] and 1:2, and a functional criterion defined as the proportion of narrower arteries at ≤10% of the total volume of the vertebral flow. Speaking of the vertebral artery hypoplasia, it should be remembered that we refer to it only if it meets the above-mentioned criteria while maintaining the condition that it eventually connects to the spinal artery of the opposite side by forming the basilar artery. Otherwise, when, for example, one of the arteries, inclusive of an artery that initially has its normal course, leaves the canal of the transverse processes at the site different from the typical one and, finishing its course, connects to a vessel other than the contralateral vertebral artery, this is considered an aplastic artery (**Figure 3**). Most often, such a connection occurs with the posterior inferior cerebellar artery of the cerebellum, yet a merger of the occipital artery or spinal arteries is also possible.

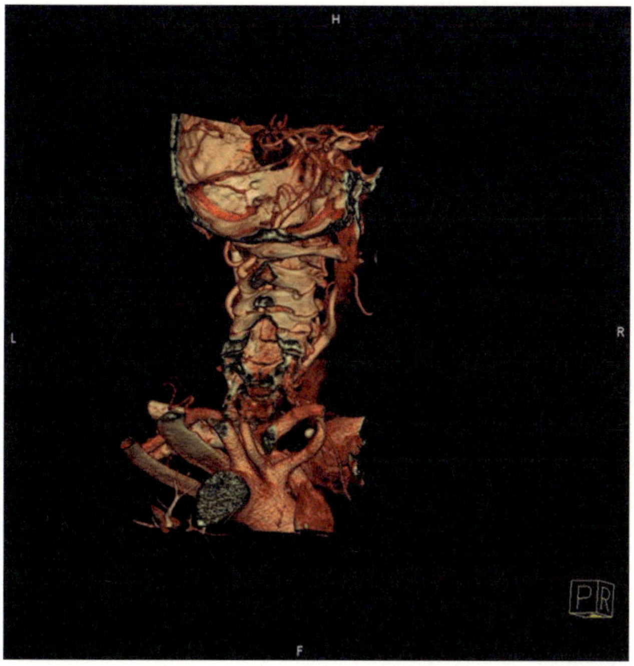

Figure 1. Angio-CT of the vertebrobasilar system vascular anomaly in the female patient. Branch-off of the right common carotid artery directly from the aortic arch with the concomitant hypoplastic right vertebral artery.

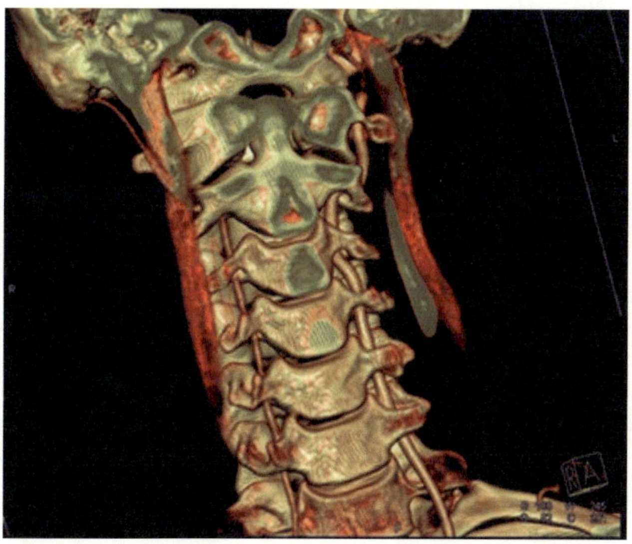

Figure 2. Angio-CT of the vertebrobasilar system vascular anomaly in the male patient. Asymmetry of the diameter of the vertebral arteries with the dominant left spinal artery.

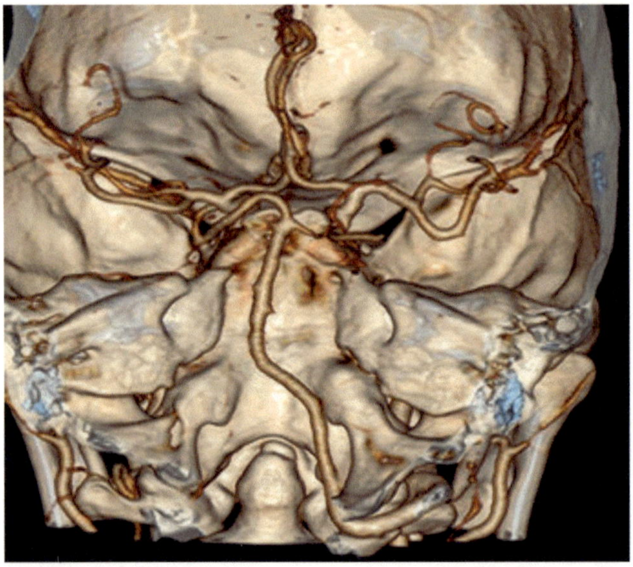

Figure 3. Angio-CT of the vertebrobasilar system vascular anomaly in the female patient. Developmental anomaly in the form of: the basilar artery that is an extension of the right vertebral artery. The left vertebral artery continues into the posterior inferior cerebellar artery.

Abnormal site of the vertebral artery branch-off is found among the typical anatomical anomalies. It can be the aortic arch—it mostly concerns the left vertebral artery (2.4–5.8% of the population), very rarely the right vertebral artery, while the simultaneous branch-off of both vertebral arteries from the aortic arch has been described in the world literature less than 10 times. Less commonly, the spinal arteries take their origin from the external or internal carotid artery whereas the left vertebral artery isolated branch-off from the common left carotid artery has been described in the literature only twice. Other anomalies of the vertebral arteries include the total lack of one of them or the double branch-off of the vertebral artery, two independent trunks of which, each originating from different vessel, then meeting in one common trunk and penetrating into the holes of the transverse processes, to complete their course in a typical manner—this type of anomaly can occur on one or both sides [16, 17].

Improper course of vertebral arteries is their another anomaly. It can be curved along the entire length of the vessel as well as in its short segment, both within the canal of the transverse processes of the cervical vertebrae and before and after leaving the canal. A staple duplication of a blood vessel can also be met which, after branching off properly splits into two trunks that run separately to merge again and complete the course by connecting to the spinal artery on the opposite side [18, 19]. Anomalies can also affect other intracranial vessels, among them the hypoplasia of the right internal carotid artery, hypoplasia of the left internal carotid artery, hypoplasia of the right common carotid artery, hypoplasia of the left subclavian artery and aplasia of the left common carotid artery. We can also meet with adult-preserved vessels of angiogenesis of the embryonic period. An analysis of the literature reveals that the above is observed especially in cases when there is abnormal flow in the vertebral, intracranial or cervical arteries due to their innate or acquired obstruction. This takes place probably because these persistent vessels constitute a connection between the system of the carotid arteries and the system of the vertebrobasilar arteries. Thus, according to their decreasing occurrence, the persistent tricuspid artery, sublingual artery, auricular artery and peri-levatorial artery can be distinguished, all taking their names from the cranial nerves along which they run [20].

The symptomatology of the presence of anomalies in intracranial vessels is very diverse and it seems to be associated with the type of existing anomalousness. The anomalies may be clinically silent and detected accidentally when performing imaging tests involving the vascular system; it may cause isolated symptoms or complex assemblies of subjective complaints in the affected person. The nature of reported complaints depends on, as mentioned above, the type of anomaly where the point is whether the given anomaly affects the capacity of the vessel in fulfilling its basic function, what the provision is of appropriate structures with blood, or it causes changes in anatomic relations resulting from the improper course or construction of the vessel which may cause adverse effects in the neighboring structures, in normal conditions not contacting with the vessel affected by the anomaly. Since the vast majority of information about the anomalies of the intracranial vessels comes from descriptions of individual cases, the search for symptoms, the occurrence of which could indicate, with a high degree of sensitivity and specificity, the existence of such a condition, is limited. Among the ailments most commonly reported in the medical literature, the paroxysmal dizziness of systemic and non-systemic nature is in the foreground. Other complaints, which may coexist or occur as isolated ailments or in groups include gait instability, nausea, double vision, presyncope/syncope, bilateral tinnitus, hearing loss, cervical radiculopathy and headaches [18, 21, 22]. Vanrietvelde et al. also described the case of a patient complaining of chronic neck pain radiating to both upper limbs for 2 months, in whom vertebral artery loop formation was revealed at the level of C4, coexisting with degenerative changes of the neighboring cervical vertebrae without imaging evidence of the spinal nerve root compression. The second case, described by the same authors, concerns the same anomaly with accompanying widening of the intervertebral foramen at the level of C4-C5, and severe torticollis with loss of sensation on the right side of the face and impaired consciousness [23].

A large and heterogeneous range of symptoms induced by the presence of the anomalies of the intracranial vessels and their not always well explained pathogenesis along with coexisting systemic diseases that may be the cause of the reported ailments, make the diagnosis of these lesions a big challenge. Therefore, it seems justified to look for more and more efficient algorithms of management, allowing at least to select a group of patients in whom diagnostic procedures will be properly targeted and more complex which finally will be the most accurate way to achieve the proper diagnosis.

1.2. Doppler ultrasound of the system of the vertebrobasilar arteries

The Doppler ultrasound is a non-invasive research modality that allows to assess the speed of blood flow in the blood vessels, which was first described by Satomura in 1959. However, the basis for its creation, that is, the discovery and definition of the Doppler phenomenon, is the merit of two physicists who had worked independently over a century before Satomura: Ch. Doppler, who in 1842 observed the effect of changing the color of light under the effect of motion in the double star system and A. Fizeau, who in 1848 described a similar phenomenon related to electromagnetic waves.

The study of Miyzaki and Kato on the measurement of the blood flow velocity in the arteries supplying the brain and in extracranial arteries was published for the first time in 1965. In 1982 Aaslid was the author of the first report about assessing the test speed of blood flow in the cerebral and intracranial vessels as well as the constructor the first measuring device. This method uses ultrasound, that is acoustic waves of frequencies exceeding the hearing range of the human ear (over 20 kHz), generated by a piezoelectric transducer. Piezoelectrics are crystals which generate an electric charge in response to applied mechanical stress and electrical fields can deform piezoelectric materials ("inverse piezoelectric effect"). The second component used in the study is the Doppler effect consisting in the change of the frequency of the wave reflected from the moving object in relation to the frequency of the wave being transmitted. Frequencies of 1–10 MHz are most commonly used for diagnostic purposes [24–26].

In the Doppler ultrasound of the blood vessels, the sound waves sent by the camera head bounce off from the blood cells flowing in the vessels, changing their frequency which is read by the ultrasound device. The change in the frequency is called the Doppler frequency and it is proportional to the speed of blood flow. In the Doppler apparatus this frequency is processed for the acoustic signal which allows to distinguish the nature and position of the vessel. Introduction of colored Doppler ultrasound has improved the identification of blood vessels and determination of the direction of blood flow. In this modality, different colors are assigned to different frequencies, depending on the direction of the moving blood cells and their speed. Red and blue colors are usually used to determine the direction of blood flow whereas shades of these colors serve to demonstrate different flow velocities. Power Doppler introduced in 1993 is an improved color Doppler ultrasonography. The difference lies in imaging of the flow by analyzing the total energy of the Doppler signal and not, as in the case of the color Doppler, the mean Doppler shift. The most important advantage of this diagnostic modality is its ability to evaluate blood vessels of smaller caliber and with low blood flow and longer segments and greater number. When evaluating the vertebral arteries, this method more precisely assesses the vessel lumen and possible atherosclerotic plaques found there.

Availability, relatively low cost, non-invasiveness and, in some cases, the possibility to supplement the information obtained from more advanced vascular imaging techniques are the advantages of Doppler ultrasonography in the diagnostics of vascular diseases. No specific preparations are needed for its implementation and the procedure itself is performed in supine position with the head slightly tilted backward and rotated in the opposite direction to the tested vessel or the head in straight position. In special cases, for example, in strong dizziness, the test may be carried out in a sitting position with the same head positioning. However, this modification should be reserved for the evaluation of the carotid but not the vertebral arteries.

In studies of the extracranial segments of the carotid and vertebral arteries vascular probes are used designed for this purpose of the footprint length not exceeding 45 mm. Their frequency should range from 5–7 to 8–12 MHz. An exception to the rule may be the use of a convex-type probe with a lower frequency of 3–5 MHz in cases of the soft tissue thickness above the average and in difficult test conditions. However, it should be remembered that, due to its lower frequency, there is no possibility of a detailed assessment of atherosclerotic lesions.

Nevertheless, when using color presentation, it is possible to evaluate the vessel course, its diameter and blood flow velocity.

According to the standards of the Polish Ultrasound Society, the examination starts with an overall assessment of the topography of blood vessels, imaging in the transverse plane, from the top of the supraclavicular area to the angles of the mandible. The main part of the procedure is carried out in long-axis view relative to the course the vessel. The following are assessed: the intima-media complex, possible atherosclerotic plaques and stenoses, both morphologically and hemodynamically. Another important part of the test is the measurement of the blood flow velocity performed in the blood stream axis inside the vessels in pre-defined locations. For the common carotid artery, it is its middle section at least 2 cm from the carotid sinus. The assessment of the internal carotid artery is carried about 1 cm above the bulb and in the external carotid artery about 1 cm above its branch-off. Measurements of the blood flow velocity in the vertebral arteries are performed in the V1 and/or V2 sections. Normal values of the blood flow velocity in individual vessels are shown in **Table 1**. When interpreting the study results the physiological decrease of the speed of the blood flow in the intracranial vessels which appears with age should be considered. These changes affect at most the common carotid arteries and subclavian arteries and, to a lesser extent, the vertebral arteries.

The cerebral arteries are examined using a 2-MHz frequency ultrasound probe applied to the so-called "acoustic windows". The acoustic windows are natural holes or thinner regions of the skull, in general there are four acoustic windows described: the transtemporal window, the transorbital window, submandibular window and suboccipital window. The basilar and the vertebral arteries in the intracranial section are assessed through the suboccipital window. The identification is made on the basis of the depth of the vessel position and the direction of the blood flow in its lumen. The basilar artery is evaluated at the depth of 80–120 mm and the direction of the blood flow is opposite to the position of the probe and the mean peak flow is 0.39 m/s. The intracranial segments of the vertebral arteries (VA) are assessed at a depth of 60–70 mm, and the mean peak flow is 0.36 m/s [26].

Numerous studies justify the use of the transcranial and classic Doppler in the assessment of the vertebrobasilar function [27–29]. In cases of a high degree of carotid stenosis (> 90%), the Power Doppler modality is a good supplementation of magnetic resonance imaging with contrast, which may in these cases yield false positive results [30]. AbuRahma et al. report the superiority of the Duplex Doppler over arteriography in the evaluation of heterogeneous atherosclerotic plaque with the average degree of carotid artery stenosis. It is also an effective tool in the diagnostics and monitoring of the treatment efficacy of the vertebral artery dissection. The Doppler ultrasound supplemented by angio-MR and angio-CT examinations is a

Vessel tested	Peak systolic velocity (m/s)	End-diastolic velocity (m/s)
Common carotid artery	0.8–1.2	0.1–0.3
Internal carotid artery	0.8–1.2	≤ 0.3
External carotid artery	0.8–1.2	≤ 0.25
Vertebral artery	<0.6	0.05–0.2

Table 1. The normal range of the blood flow velocity in the intracranial vessels in Doppler ultrasonography (m/s).

reliable tool in detecting flow disturbances in the middle cerebral artery and the vertebral arteries, which cause tinnitus [31]. It is also used in traumatology and is comparable with arteriography in detecting traumatic changes in cervical vessels.

The more and more perfect ultrasound technique allows to limit the number of invasive tests required for performing vascular examinations, thus reducing the patient's exposure to complications associated with them.

2. Overview

Our previous studies [9] concerning the analysis of the frequency and types of anatomical anomalies of the cranial arteries, i.e. vertebral and carotid arteries, in patients with dizziness and impaired hearing, demonstrated that the most common anatomical anomaly of cranial arteries was hypoplasia of the right vertebral artery, occurring in 58.7% of cases, of which 51.7% were women and 6.9% men; hypoplasia of the left vertebral artery, occurring in 24.7% of the study group, of which 13.8% were women and 10.3% men; hypoplasia of the right internal carotid artery found in 3.4% of women, and of the left internal carotid artery in 6.8% of cases, 3.4% in women and 3.4% in men; and hypoplasia of the right common carotid artery was reported in 3.4% of men, while critical stenosis of the left subclavian artery with subclavian steal syndrome was observed in 3.4% of women. Although the most common symptom occurring in these patients was tinnitus, the most frequent cause found in patients admitted to the Department for diagnosis was dizziness, possibly because the patients found it more disturbing.

In the case of anatomical anomalies it is difficult to make any suggestions as to the nature of abnormalities without carrying out imaging tests.

The diagnostic procedure to detect anatomical abnormalities in the cranial arteries generally starts with vascular ultrasound. Blood flow disorders observed on the ultrasound should be further verified by contrast CTA or MRA to evaluate the morphology of the artery [2].

However, the diagnostics of vertigo does not always involve contrast CT angiography of the cranial arteries. In our study, the ultrasound of the vertebrobasilar system showed no abnormalities in the blood flow velocity, a vascular anomaly being only suggested by pathological blood flow velocity on ultrasound after applying the neck torsion test.

Normally, the unpaired basilar artery is formed by both vertebral arteries merging on the clivus of the occipital bone. In turn, the labyrinthine artery is a paired thin vessel originating from the middle section of the basilar artery or from the anterior inferior cerebellar artery which runs laterally along with the atrio-cochlear nerve and enters the internal auditory canal to vascularize the inner ear structures. The anterior inferior cerebellar artery is a paired vessel originating from the lower part of the basilar artery, finally merging with the posterior inferior cerebellar artery.

In the presented case, the basilar artery was an extension of the right vertebral artery, and the left atrophic vertebral artery extended into the posterior inferior cerebellar artery whereas the labyrinthine artery originated bilaterally from the basilar artery.

The described vascular anomaly, osteochondrosis of the C4/C5 and hyperlipidemia present in the patient resulted in mixed-type vertigo with decreased excitability of the labyrinth on the affected side (anomaly) due to insufficient blood supply to the inner ear and the lack of vascular compensation of the vertebral artery on the other side.

The treatment of diagnosed anatomical anomalies in adults is usually conservative and depends on coexisting disorders. Surgical treatment in the case of disorders of blood supply to the central nervous system caused by anomalous cranial vessels includes implantation of stents, arterial anastomosis and vascular bypass.

Conservative treatment and implementation of motor rehabilitation resulted in a very good therapeutic effect in the patient.

Author details

Jurek Olszewski* and Piotr Niewiadomski

*Address all correspondence to: jurek.olszewski@umed.lodz.pl

Department of Otolaryngology, Laryngological Oncology, Audiology and Phoniatrics, Medical University of Lodz, Lodz, Poland

References

[1] Acar M, Degirmenci B, Yucel A, Albayrak R, Haktanir A. An evaluation of internal carotid artery and cerebral blood flow volume using color duplex sonography in patients with vertebral artery hypoplasia. European Journal of Radiology. 2005;**53**:450-453

[2] Drobisz AT, Herfurt W. The vertebrobasilar syndrome and other pathologies of vertebral arteries by Doppler ultrasound. Udar Mózgu. 2001;**3**(1):35-41

[3] Olszewski J, Majak J, Pietkiewicz P, Łuszcz C, Repetowski M. The association between positional veretebral and basilar artery flow lesion and prevalence of vertigo in patients with cervical spondylosis. Otolaryngology—Head and Neck Surgery. 2006;**134**:680-684

[4] Poona M, Singla RK, Sharma T. Incidence of anomalous origins of vertebral artery—Anatomical study and clinical significance. Journal of Clinical and Diagnostic Research. 2010;**4**:2626-2631

[5] Mysior M, Majos A, Grzelak P, Szubert W, Stachowiak S, Stefańczyk L. Hypoplasia of the vertebral artery and symptoms of vertebrobasilar insufficiency in menopause. Przegląd Menopauzalny. 2007;**5**:298-302

[6] Paksoy Y, Vatansev H, Seker M, Ustun ME, Buyukmumcu M, Akpinar Z. Congenital morphological abnormalities of the distal vertebral arteries (CMADVA) and their relationship with vertigo and dizziness. Medical Science Monitor. 2004;**10**(7):316-323

[7] Soustiel JF, Shik V, Shreiber R, Tavor Y, Goldsher D. Basilar vasospasm diagnosis: Investigation of a modified "Lindegaard index" based on imaging studies and blood velocity measurements of the basilar artery. Stroke. 2002;**33**(1):72-77

[8] Strupp M, Planck JH, Arbusow V, Steiger J, Bruckmann H, Brandt T. Rotational vertebral artery occlusion syndrome with vertigo due to "labyrinthine excitation". Neurology. 2000; **28**(6):1376-1379

[9] Miłoński J, Kuśmierczyk K, Mielczarek M, Niewiadomski P, Olszewski J. Anatomical anomalies of cranial arteries in patients with vertigo and hearing disorders. Otolaryngologia polska. 2013;**67**(20):77-81

[10] Li W, Feng Y, Lu W, Xie X, Xiong Z, Jing Z, Cai X, Huang L. Evaluating the morphological changes of intracranial arteries and whole-brain perfusion in undetermined isolated vertigo. Journal of the Neurological Sciences. 2016;**370**(15):70-77

[11] Lee J, Park S, Kim H, Kim M, Park B, Kim J. Vulnerability of the vestibular organs to transient ischemia: Implications for isolated vascular vertigo. Neuroscience Letters. 2014; **558**:180-185

[12] Choi KD, Lee H, Kim JS. Ischemic syndromes causing dizziness and vertigo. Handbook of Clinical Neurology. 2016;**137**:317-340

[13] Skultéty Szárazová A, Bartels E, Turčáni P. Vertebral artery hypoplasia and the posterior circulation stroke. Perspectives in Medicine. 2012;**1**(1–12):198-202

[14] Wells D, Petersen D. Prevalence of intraforaminal vertebral artery loops. The Spine Journal. 2010;**10**(9):69-70

[15] Faisal MS, Hurley A, Buckley O, Tierney S. Kommerell's diverticulum, right-sided aortic arch and a hypoplastic left vertebral artery arising from the left common carotid artery. Journal of Vascular Surgery. 2014;**60**(4):1059-1064

[16] Khan S, Cloud GC, Kerry S, Markus HS. Imaging of vertebral artery stenosis: A systematic review. Journal of Neurology, Neurosurgery, and Psychiatry. 2007;**78**:1218-1225

[17] Troutman DA, Bicking GK, Madden NJ, Domer GS. Aberrant origin of left vertebral artery. Journal of Vascular Surgery. 2013;**58**(6):1670-1676

[18] Al-Okaili R, Schwartz ED. Bilateral aortic origins of the vertebral arteries with right vertebral artery arising distal to left subclavian artery: Case report. Surgical Neurology. 2007;**67**(2):174-176

[19] Min J-H, Lee Y-S. Transcranial Doppler ultrasonographic evaluation of vertebral artery hypoplasia and aplasia. Journal of the Neurological Sciences. 2007;**260**:183-187

[20] Mordasini P, Schmidt F, Schroth G, Remonda L. Asymmetrical bilateral duplication of the extracranial vertebral arteries: Report of a unique case. European Journal of Radiology Extra. 2008;**67**:91-94

[21] Back JD, Herzog RJ, Lutz GE. A rare anomaly of the course of the vertebral artery. The Spine Journal. 2011;**11**(7):681-682

[22] Hong-Tao Z, Shu-Ling Z, Dao-Pei Z. Two case reports of bilateral vertebral artery tortuosity and spiral twisting in vascular vertigo. BMC Neurology. 2014;**14**:14-19

[23] Cao YH, Zhang GY, Cheng SQ, Han JL, Zhao G. Proatlantal intersegmental artery with absence of the common carotid artery. Clinical Neurology and Neurosurgery. 2011;**113**(3): 245-246

[24] Yamanaka T, Sawai Y, Hosoi H. Bilateral subclavian steal syndrome with vertigo. Auris Nasus Larynx. 2014;**41**(3):307-309

[25] Chibbaro S, Mirone G, Yasuda M, Marsella M, Di Emidio P, George B. Vertebral artery loop—A cause of cervical radiculopathy: Review article. World Neurosurgery. 2012;(3–4): **78**, 375.e11-375.e13

[26] Rocha MD, Nakao BH, Manoel EM, Moussalem GF, Ganança FF. Vertebral artery dissection: An important differentia diagnosis of vertigo. Brazilian Journal of Otorhinolaryngology 2015; Available online

[27] Terenzi T. Transcranial sonography and vertebrobasilar insufficiency. Journal of Manipulative and Physiological Therapeutics. 2002;**25**(3):180-183

[28] Harper C, Cardullo PA, Weyman AK, Patterson RB. Transcranial Doppler ultrasonography of the basilar artery in patients with retrograde vertebral artery flow. Journal of Vascular Surgery. 2008;**48**(4):859-864

[29] Wang W, Zhu LY, Shi JH. Cerebral blood flow and hemodynamics in patients with dizziness resulting from central nervous system disorders. Di Yi Jun Yi Da Xue Bau. 2003;**23**(4):384-386

[30] Clevert A, Johnson T, Michaely H, Jung EM, Flach PM, Strautz TI, Clevert A, Reiser M, Schoenberg SO. High-grade stenoses of the internal carotid artery: Comparison of high-resolution contrast enhanced 3D MRA, duplex sonography and power Doppler imaging. European Journal of Radiology. 2006;**60**(3):379-386

[31] Cardona P, Quesada H, Cano L, Campdelacreu J, Escrig A, Mora P, Rubio F. Transcranial and cervical duplex: A feasible approach to the diagnosis of pulsatile tinnitus. Perspectives in Medicine. 2012;**1**(1–12):446-448

Chapter 2

Carotid Artery Stenting in High-Risk Patients for Stenting

Mohamed Khaled Elewa

Additional information is available at the end of the chapter

http://dx.doi.org/10.5772/intechopen.82019

Abstract

Certain subgroups of patients are at higher risk for CAS. The identification of those patients could improve the decision-making and hence the outcome. This chapter covers factors that are associated with poor outcome during CAS based on the previously reported literature: (1) CAS in female patients, (2) CAS in octogenarians, (3) CAS in patients with difficult aortic arch configuration (type II, III, and bovine arch), (4) CAS in patients who have tortuous common carotid artery (CCA), angulated internal carotid artery (ICA) origin, and/or angulated distal ICA, (5) CAS in high-grade carotid stenosis, (6) CAS for long lesions (≥15 mm), (7) CAS for ostial-centered lesions, (8) CAS in the presence of calcified aortic arch and/or heavily calcified lesions, (9) CAS in the presence of contralateral carotid occlusion, (10) CAS in the presence of vertebral artery occlusion and/or stenosis, and (11) CAS in chronic kidney disease patients.

Keywords: carotid artery stenting, high-risk patients, female gender, octogenarian, difficult arch, tortuous common carotid, tortuous internal carotid, high-grade stenosis, long lesion, ostial stenosis, contralateral occlusion, vertebral artery occlusion, vertebral artery stenosis, chronic kidney

1. Introduction

The term "high-risk patients" was used extensively in the literature when talking about carotid intervention, unfortunately, with inconsistent meaning. Here, this term refers to patients at higher risk during carotid artery stenting (CAS).

The term high-risk carotid artery stenting raises an important question: is there any population at higher risk during carotid artery stenting? The identification of population at higher risk during

CAS could improve the decision-making, regarding patient selection and the used technique. Periprocedural risk of CAS is influenced by patient, device, technique, and operator-related factors. The outcome of CAS in those patients should be defined with respect to standard carotid endarterectomy (CEA), particularly in low-surgical risk patients and high-CAS risk patients.

2. CAS in subgroups at higher risk

2.1. CAS in female patients

The prevalence of carotid artery stenosis (>50%) in elderly females was 6% (8% for males), based on the data that were derived from the American Vascular Association screening program in 2002–2003 [1]. Many gender differences were reported in literature regarding the anatomy, physiology, and atherosclerotic pathology of carotid arteries. The carotid arteries in females have higher velocities in comparison to males [2], with higher outflow/inflow ratio. The atherosclerotic disease in females tends to affect the common carotid artery rather than the proximal internal carotid artery [3]. Meanwhile, the carotid atherosclerotic plaque in females carries more stable characteristics [4].

CEA is a valid option in preventing complications of carotid stenosis. However, the value of CEA in women with asymptomatic disease is questionable. CAS has emerged as an alternative to CEA in selected patients. Several trials [5–7] have compared CEA and CAS; unfortunately, they were not designed for subgroup analysis as regards gender effect on the outcome, especially in asymptomatic patients.

The large trials (the VA cooperative trial, the asymptomatic carotid atherosclerosis study (ACAS), and the asymptomatic carotid surgery trial (ACST)) approving CEA in asymptomatic patients either did not perform subgroup analysis for female patients or did not find significant effect in women. The VA cooperative trial studied males only.

The ACAS showed a 66% [95% confidence interval (CI), 36–82%] 5 years relative stroke risk reduction for males, on the other hand, statistically insignificant risk reduction for females 17% (95% CI, −96 to 65%) [8]. This difference was explained with higher perioperative rates of death or stroke seen in females than males (3.6 vs. 1.7%; $P = 0.12$), while the ACST showed 4.1% long-term nonperioperative risk reduction of stroke for females. The benefit was marginal when compared with perioperative risk of stroke or death (3.8%) [9].

The carotid revascularization endarterectomy versus stent trial (CREST) did not show sex difference as regards treatment effect [10, 11]. However, women had showed significantly higher perioperative stroke rate with CAS than CEA (5.5 vs. 1.7%; $P = 0.01$). The rates of myocardial infarction (MI) for women were equivalent for both CAS and CEA (1.5 vs. 1.7%, respectively; $P = 0.81$).

The availability of comprehensive medical treatment and CAS as alternative options to CEA added to the complexity of the decision-making in asymptomatic females. Further research is needed in this area.

2.2. CAS in octogenarians

The studies, which have validated CEA for stroke prevention in symptomatic and asymptomatic carotid stenosis patients, have excluded high-risk patients for surgery (including octogenarians) [8, 12, 13]. On the other hand, other smaller studies have shown safety of CEA in octogenarians [14–19].

The CREST trial reported 12% 30-day rate of stroke and death among octogenarians [20]. Kastrup et al. reported 10% rate of stroke and death among symptomatic patients and 13% among asymptomatic patients >75 years [21]. Stanziale and his colleagues reported 8% 30-day stroke among octogenarians [22].

In a meta-analysis for three randomized controlled trials, the treatment effect was modified by age in the CAS group (12 vs. 5.8% in patients <70 years) [23].

The high rate of stroke in octogenarians is partially assumed to unfavorable anatomy which precludes safe navigation; this was reported in several studies [24–27]. This includes aortic arch elongation, aortic calcification, ostial stenosis, and vessel tortuosity. Lam and his colleagues [26] assessed 133 CAS patients for the anatomic characteristics that affect the feasibility of CAS. They found increased incidence of unfavorable anatomical characteristics among octogenarians in comparison with younger patients; arch elongation (82 vs. 56%, P = 0.008), arch calcification (59 vs. 30%, P = 0.003), common carotid artery origin stenosis (47 vs. 22%, P = 0.006), common carotid artery tortuosity (70 vs. 38%, P = 0.0009), and internal carotid artery tortuosity (74 vs. 50%, P = 0.019). It has been suggested that with correcting for complex anatomy, old age was no longer a predictor for poor outcome [26, 28–30]. Unfortunately, other age-related factors may increase the risk in such age group. Specific comorbidities such as congestive heart failure, aortic stenosis, and contralateral carotid stenosis are more common among octogenarians [20, 22, 27, 31, 32]. On the other hand, different mechanisms such as emboli, hypoperfusion, and neuronal susceptibility in elderly contribute to increased risk for CAS [33].

Werner and his colleagues reported a 10-fold increase in death among octogenarians compared to younger patients [27]; they attribute their finding to high incidence of symptomatic aortic stenosis among octogenarians. Three of 12 patients with this problem died before discharge; death occurred only in preoperatively decompensated patients. The safety of CAS in severe aortic stenosis patients was assessed in small cohort (52 patient); the 30-day death rate was 6%. Noteworthy, all patients in that cohort were hemodynamically stable prior to CAS [34].

Despite the higher CAS periprocedural risk, surprisingly, octogenarians have fewer comorbidities [35]. We think that good selection of octogenarian CAS candidates can minimize the perioperative risk. A more comprehensive preoperative assessment is needed in such group of patients.

2.3. CAS in patients with difficult aortic arch configuration (type II, III, and bovine arch)

Aortic arch type is a key in CAS success. Difficult aortic arch is associated with repeated aggressive manipulation, which may generate emboli. Nevertheless, unfavorable aortic arch configuration may impede guiding catheter or long sheath insertion. Faggioli and his colleagues reported that the proximal tortuosity (difficult aortic arch due to arterial elongation) was associated with technical failure [36]. Type of arch was found to contribute to higher stroke rates in six of the seven studies. [21, 25, 27, 37–39]. Wimmer and his colleagues [37] reported that type II and III arches were predictors of stroke following carotid stenting, whereas Werner et al. [27] found the same with bovine arches. Dumont et al. [39] demonstrated that unfavorable arch anatomy, namely a target vessel taking an acute angle off the arch, was a predictor of perioperative stroke risk. In fact, in certain studies, type III aortic arch was contraindicated for CAS [40].

The carotid revascularization endarterectomy versus stenting trial 2 (CREST-2) study will compare outcomes in asymptomatic carotid stenosis patients randomized to best medical treatment (BMT) versus CEA plus BMT versus CAS plus BMT, and patients will be excluded from undergoing CAS if they have a type III arch, severely angled or tortuous innominate artery or CCA, or a severely calcified aortic arch [41].

Radial, brachial, or direct carotid access may be used as alternative for femoral in this subgroup of patients. Alternative access may increase the technical success rate and decrease the perioperative risk of complication.

2.4. CAS in patients who have tortuous common carotid artery (CCA), angulated internal carotid artery (ICA) origin, and/or angulated distal ICA

Tortuous carotid is found on ~16% of cerebral angiograms [42]. Carotid tortuosity represents a challenge in patients undergoing CAS. Wimmer et al. [37], Faggioli et al. [36], and Fanous et al. [43] found that tortuosity of the CCA and proximal ICA were correlated with both technical failure and increased risk of complications. The periprocedural risk significantly increased in a study of 262 patients with symptomatic carotid artery stenosis when the angulation between the ICA and the CCA exceeded 60° [44]. Similarly, the stroke risk was correlated with severe tortuosity of the CCA and significant angulation of the ICA origin in an unselected population of 751 patients who underwent 833 CAS procedures [27]. In fact, several authors were forced to abort CAS procedures secondary to severe ICA tortuosity [26, 45, 46]. Myouchin reported that among 31 symptomatic and asymptomatic carotid artery stenosis patients, successful stenting was not possible in two (6.5%) patients because of severe carotid tortuosity (angles of 60° and 73°) [47].

An anatomically difficult distal landing zone not only makes deployment of protection devices more difficult but also makes the retrieval of these devices more challenging [43, 48, 49]. Reimers et al. [50] reported that the distal EPD could not be advanced beyond the lesion in 10 patients owing to high degree of distal ICA tortuosity and lesion severity in a series of 753 patients who underwent 808 CAS procedures. Fanous et al. [43] reported that despite the successful deployment and retrieval of distal EPD in all cases, the presence of hostile anatomy for the deployment of distal EPD was correlated with increased periprocedural risk among 221 symptomatic patients who underwent CAS.

2.5. CAS in high-grade carotid stenosis

Critical stenosis (>85%) was previously considered by some authors as a contraindication for CAS [40, 42]. Earlier, critical stenosis was technically challenging, as it impeded the safe advancement of distal EPD [43, 44]. With improvement of the available endovascular devices, stenting of such lesion is no more challenging except for subtotal occlusion (99% stenosis). Subtotal occlusion was associated with increased perioperative risk [43, 52].

2.6. CAS for long lesions (≥15 mm)

The American Heart Association/American College of Cardiology defines lesion length as the distance from the definite proximal to distal shoulder of the lesion in the projection of the best elongation of the stenosis. Only the portion of stenosis that was ≥50% was quantified [42].

Long lesions (≥15 mm) carry higher risk of poor outcome, even in the presence of cerebral protection [37]. The periprocedural stroke rate in those patients group was 17 versus 2.1% in other patients. Also, they were more prone to 30-day adverse events (19.1 vs. 3.4% in other patients) [25].

It seems that proximal protection devices may be more suitable in those patients with long lesions. Saini and his colleagues reported that patients with carotid lesions >10 mm length who underwent CAS with proximal protection devices showed a trend of better safety outcomes including perioperative stroke than patients with distal protection devices [53].

2.7. CAS for ostial-centered lesions

The definition of ostial lesions should be limited to those lesions with maximum stenosis at the ostium of the ICA.

Difficult wire engagement and hemodynamic instability are more common to occur with ostial lesions [43]. They are associated with higher rate of stroke and cardiac complications [44–46].

Sayeed and his colleagues reported that patients with ostial lesions have higher incidence of periprocedural stroke (7.1 vs. 1.8% in patients without ostial lesions). The rates of 30-day adverse events were also higher in those patients (9.1 vs. 2.9%) [25].

2.8. CAS in the presence of calcified aortic arch and/or heavily calcified lesions

Extensive calcification either concentric carotid calcification or aortic arch calcification was associated with increased perioperative risk [47–49]. They were considered a contraindication for CAS in certain studies [50, 51].

On the other hand, Tsutsumi and his colleagues reported the feasibility of CAS in near-total circumferential calcified lesions, with no reported morbidity or mortality [54].

Bazan and his colleagues studied 94 patients. They found that the patient ≥75-years old have significantly more aortic arch calcification than younger patients. They advised for preprocedural assessment of arch calcification as method for CAS risk stratification [28].

Kastrup and his colleagues studied 62 symptomatic patients (49 aged <80 years; 13 aged >80 years) who underwent CAS. They found that octogenarians had a significantly higher incidence of severe aortic arch calcification (54 vs. 14%, P < 0.01). A severe aortic arch calcification was found to be a predictor for new DWI lesions inside and outside the treated territory (OR, 1.8; 95% CI, 0.99–3335; P = 0.05) [55].

2.9. CAS in the presence of contralateral carotid occlusion

Patients with CCO have bilateral carotid disease and therefore may have increased cardiovascular risk. The impaired collateral system and the perioperative hemodynamic changes may contribute in increased risk during carotid intervention in those patients.

The range of incidence of contralateral carotid occlusion (CCO) among CEA patients was 6–10% [56].

The North American symptomatic carotid endarterectomy trial (NASCET) [57, 58] and two meta-analysis [59, 60] showed that the contralateral carotid occlusion was a predictor of poor outcome after ipsilateral CEA. The presence of contralateral carotid artery occlusion was considered as high-risk criteria for CEA in many trials [5, 37]. On the other hand, Rockman and his colleagues reviewed previous studies and concluded that the presence of CCO does not increase the CEA perioperative risk [61]. Kretz and his colleagues identified one study in their meta-analysis that reported different outcome for patients with and without CCO after CEA [62]. Many large center trials have reported excellent outcome after CEA in patients with CCO [63–66]. A retrospective analysis of CEA operative data in patients with CCO and/or vertebral artery occlusion (VAO) revealed that the presence of CCO increases the need for carotid shunt during CEA but did not increase the perioperative risk. [67] Worth to know, among CEA patients who had CCO, the procedural outcome was not affected using shunts [56].

Halm and his colleagues reported that contralateral carotid stenosis >50% was independent predictor for stroke after CEA [68].

Yang and his colleagues retrospectively analyzed the data of 698 CEA patients and 455 CAS patients. They reported that the CCO was associated with higher rate of early symptomatic neurological complication (ESNC) but not stroke alone in CEA patients only. Vertebral artery occlusion either unilateral or bilateral was not associated with increased risk of ESNC or stroke in CEA or CAS patients [69].

The posterior part of circle of Willis provides collateral supply to contralateral hemisphere during carotid clamping in patients with CCO. The CCO patients with incomplete posterior part of circle of Willis are at higher risk of cerebral ischemia during carotid clamping [70].

Elective CAS in patients with contralateral high-grade carotid stenosis or occlusion was not associated with poor neurological outcome [71–73]. On the other side, based on the carotid artery revascularization and endarterectomy (CARE) registry, Mercado and his colleagues reported increased risk of early post CAS stroke, myocardial infarction, or death in CCO patients [74].

Ricotta and his colleagues evaluated 1128 CAS and 666 CEA patients with CCO. They concluded that the benefit of lower periprocedural risk CEA is lost in patients with CCO because of increased stroke rates in those patients. CAS periprocedural risk was not affected by the presence of CCO regardless of the symptomatic state [56].

In patients with CCO, CAS has theoretical advantages over CEA, of short carotid occlusion duration and the lack of general anesthesia. It is important to know that CCO is one of the factors that identify patients at high risk for CEA and qualify them for reimbursement of CAS according to the Centers for Medicare & Medicaid Services (CMS). We think that in the presence of CCO or contralateral high-grade carotid stenosis, CAS should be encouraged over CEA.

2.10. CAS in the presence of vertebral artery occlusion or stenosis

In patients with unilateral carotid occlusion, Nicolau and his colleagues observed increase in the peak systolic velocity and blood volume in vertebral artery [75].

Severe vertebral artery stenosis (>80%) was associated with increased 30 days risk of stroke or death in CEA patients [76]. On the other hand, Yang and his colleagues found that unilateral or bilateral vertebral artery occlusion (VAO) was not a risk factor for early symptomatic neurological complication or postoperative stroke in CEA or CAS patients [69].

Currently, no special recommendation regarding cases with vertebra-basilar occlusive disease, yet in some cases, the author may prefer CAS to avoid the effect of general anesthesia and temporal carotid clamping, which may be dangerous.

2.11. CAS in chronic kidney disease patients

Patient is defined to have chronic kidney disease (CKD) once the estimated glomerular filtration rate (eGFR) is less than 60 mL/min/1.73 m^2. Once the patient has renal failure that necessitates dialysis, he is considered to have end-stage renal disease (ESRD). CKD patients are at higher risk for ischemic stroke than general population [77]. Extracranial carotid artery disease is a common comorbidity in CKD patients [78].

The available data on the outcome of CEA or CAS in those patients are scarce. All CKD patients are at high surgical risk [79]. AbuRahma and his colleagues studied the effect of CKD of CEA outcome and concluded that the patients with moderate to severe CKD (GFR <60) had increased risk of stroke or death and, that CEA should not be used as alternative for CAS in CKD patients [80]. Tarakji and his colleagues retrospectively reviewed the outcomes of CEA in CKD patients including hemodialysis patients. They classified

CKD patients into three groups according to serum creatinine level into: normal renal function, 121 patients with mild renal impairment (serum creatinine 1.6–2.9 mg/dL), and 23 patients with severe renal impairment (serum creatinine >2.9 mg/dL or requiring hemodialysis). In patients with mild renal impairment, the incidence of stroke, MI, and death were 2.4, 9.0, and 4.9%, respectively. The figures were higher in patient with severe renal impairment; incidence of stroke, MI, and death was 9.5, 4.7, and 9.5%, respectively [81]. Rigdon and his colleagues assessed the outcome of CEA in CKD patients (21 patient with mild renal impairment and 7 patients with severe renal impairment). Patients with mild renal impairment had the same perioperative outcome of patients with normal kidney function. Patients with severe renal impairment had higher rate of stroke and death (43%) [82].

Donahue and his colleagues studied 126 CKD patients who underwent CAS for the risk of acute kidney injury (AKI) and 30 days major adverse events. AKI occurred in 26 patients (21%) and mostly caused by hemodynamic depression (mainly hypotension). AKI was associated with a higher rate of 30 days major adverse events [83].

Chronic kidney disease (CKD) was an independent predictor of CAS periprocedural complications and long-term disability [35, 37, 84]. On the other hand, a care registry analysis showed that CKD was not an independent predictor for early outcome [85].

Saw et al. studied the outcome of CAS in CKD patients. They reported that the presence of CKD was associated with higher combined endpoints of MI, stroke, and mortality at 7 days (4.1%) and 6 months (8.8%) [84].

Adil and his colleagues retrospectively reviewed the United States nationwide inpatient sample data files from 2005 to 2011 for the outcome of end-stage renal disease (ESRD) and CKD patients who underwent CAS or CEA. They reported that 43,875 CEA were performed in CKD patients, 3888 (8.8%) of them were ESRD patients. ESRD patients were associated with higher rates of in-hospital mortality (odds ratio (OR) 4.3, 95% confidence interval (CI) 2.1–9.0; $P \leq 0.0001$) and moderate to severe disability (OR 1.4, 95% CI 1.1–1.8; $P = 0.009$). On the other side, 8148 CKD patients underwent CAS, 693 (8.5%) of them were ESRD patients. ESRD patients were associated with higher rates of in-hospital mortality (OR 3.7, 95% CI 1.0–13.9; $P = 0.04$) and moderate to severe disability (OR 1.7, 95% CI 1.0–3.3; $P = 0.05$). No significant difference was found between both the procedures in ESRD patients [86].

Unfortunately, the result of these studies cannot be generalized due to lack of power, patient selection bias, and retrospective nature of these studies. CKD patients are high-risk surgical candidates, and CAS may be advised in the author opinion.

Conflict of interest

There are no conflicts of interests.

Author details

Mohamed Khaled Elewa

Address all correspondence to: m_khaled79@med.asu.edu.eg

Department of Neurology, Ain Shams University Hospitals, Cairo, Egypt

References

[1] Cheanvechai V, Harthun NL, Graham LM, Freischlag JA, Gahtan V. Incidence of peripheral vascular disease in women: Is it different from that in men? The Journal of Thoracic and Cardiovascular Surgery. 2004;**127**:314-317

[2] Comerota AJ, Salles-Cunha SX, Daoud Y, Jones L, Beebe HG. Gender differences in blood velocities across carotid stenoses. Journal of Vascular Surgery. 2004;**40**:939-944

[3] Schulz UG, Rothwell PM. Sex differences in carotid bifurcation anatomy and the distribution of atherosclerotic plaque. Stroke. 2001;**32**:1525-1531

[4] Hellings WE, Pasterkamp G, Verhoeven BA, De Kleijn DP, De Vries JP, Seldenrijk KA, et al. Gender-associated differences in plaque phenotype of patients undergoing carotid endarterectomy. Journal of Vascular Surgery. 2007;**45**:289-297

[5] Yadav JS, Wholey MH, Kuntz RE, Fayad P, Katzen BT, Mishkel GJ, et al. Protected carotid-artery stenting versus endarterectomy in high-risk patients. The New England Journal of Medicine. 2004;**351**:1493-1501

[6] SPACE Collaborative Group, Ringleb PA, Allenberg J, Bruckmann H, Brückmann H, Eckstein HH, et al. 30 day results from the SPACE trial of stent-protected angioplasty versus carotid endarterectomy in symptomatic patients: A randomized non-inferiority trial. Lancet. 2006;**368**:1239-1247

[7] Mas JL, Chatellier G, Beyssen B, et al. Endarterectomy versus stenting in patients with symptomatic severe carotid stenosis. The New England Journal of Medicine. 2006;**355**(16):1660-1671

[8] Executive Committee for the Asymptomatic Carotid Atherosclerosis Study. Endarterectomy for asymptomatic carotid artery stenosis. JAMA. 1995;**273**:1421-1428

[9] Halliday A, Mansfield A, Marro J, Peto C, Peto R, Potter J, et al. Prevention of disabling and fatal strokes by successful carotid endarterectomy in patients without recent neurological symptoms: Randomized controlled trial. Lancet. 2004;**363**:1491-1502

[10] Howard VJ, Lutsep HL, Mackey A, Demaerschalk BM, Sam AD 2nd, Gonzales NR, et al. Influence of sex on outcomes of stenting versus endarterectomy: A subgroup analysis

of the carotid revascularization endarterectomy versus stenting trial (CREST). Lancet Neurology. 2011;**10**:530-537

[11] Brott TG, Hobson RW 2nd, Howard G, Roubin GS, Clark WM, Brooks W, et al. Stenting versus endarterectomy for treatment of carotid-artery stenosis. The New England Journal of Medicine. 2010;**363**:11-23

[12] North American Symptomatic Carotid Endarterectomy Trial Collaborators. Beneficial effect of carotid endarterectomy in symptomatic patients with high-grade carotid stenosis. The New England Journal of Medicine. 1991;**325**:445-453

[13] Mayberg MR, Wilson SE, Yatsu F, Weiss DG, Messina L, Hershey LA, et al. Carotid endarterectomy and prevention of cerebral ischemia in symptomatic carotid stenosis. JAMA. 1991;**266**:3289-3294

[14] Ballotta E, Renon L, Da Giau G, Barbon B, Terranova O, Baracchini C. Octogenarians with contralateral carotid artery occlusion: A cohort at higher risk for carotid endarterectomy? Journal of Vascular Surgery. 2004;**39**:1003-1008

[15] Mozes G, Sullivan TM, Torres-Russotto DR, Bower TC, Hoskin TL, Sampaio SM, et al. Carotid endarterectomy in SAPPHIRE-eligible high-risk patients: Implications for selecting patients for carotid angioplasty and stenting. Journal of Vascular Surgery. 2004;**39**:958-966

[16] Norman PE, Semmens JB, Laurvick CL, Lawrence-Brown M. Longterm relative survival in elderly patients after carotid endarterectomy: A population-based study. Stroke. 2003;**34**:e95-e98

[17] Rockman CB, Jacobowitz GR, Adelman MA, Lamparello PJ, Gagne PJ, Landis R, et al. The benefits of carotid endarterectomy in the octogenarian: A challenge to the results of carotid angioplasty and stenting. Annals of Vascular Surgery. 2003;**17**:9-14

[18] Schneider JR, Droste JS, Schindler N, Golan JR. Carotid endarterectomy in octogenarians: Comparison with patient characteristics and outcomes in younger patients. Journal of Vascular Surgery. 2000;**31**:927-935

[19] Alamowitch S, Eliasziw M, Algra A, Meldrum H, Barnett HJ. North American symptomatic carotid endarterectomy trial (NASCET) group, risk, causes, and prevention of ischaemic stroke in elderly patients with symptomatic internal-carotid-artery stenosis. Lancet. 2001;**357**:1154-1160

[20] Hobson RW 2nd, Howard VJ, Roubin GS, Brott TG, Ferguson RD. Carotid artery stenting is associated with increased complications in octogenarians: 30-day stroke and death rates in the CREST lead-in phase. Journal of Vascular Surgery. 2004;**40**:1106-1111

[21] Kastrup A, Schulz JB, Raygrotzki S, Groschel K, Ernemann U. Comparison of angioplasty and stenting with cerebral protection versus endarterectomy for treatment of internal carotid artery stenosis in elderly patients. Journal of Vascular Surgery. 2004;**40**:945-951

[22] Stanziale SF, Marone LK, Boules RN, Brimmeier JA, Hill K, Makaroun MS, et al. Carotid artery stenting in octogenarians is associated with increased adverse outcomes. Journal of Vascular Surgery. 2006;**43**:297-304

[23] Bonati LH, Dobson J, Algra A, Branchereau A, Chatellier G, Fraedrich G, et al. Short-term outcome after stenting versus endarterectomy for symptomatic carotid stenosis: A preplanned meta-analysis of individual patient data. Lancet. 2010;**376**:1062-1073

[24] Madhwal S, Rajagopal V, Bhatt DL, Bajzer CT, Whitlow P, Kapadia SR. Predictors of difficult carotid stenting as determined by aortic arch angiography. The Journal of Invasive Cardiology. 2008;**20**:200-204

[25] Sayeed S, Stanziale SF, Wholey MH, Makaroun MS. Angiographic lesion characteristics can predict adverse outcomes after carotid artery stenting. Journal of Vascular Surgery. 2008;**47**:81-87

[26] Lam RC, Lin SC, DeRubertis B, Hynecek R, Kent KC, Faries PL. The impact of increasing age on anatomic factors affecting carotid angioplasty and stenting. Journal of Vascular Surgery. 2007;**45**(5):875-880

[27] Werner M, Bausback Y, Bräunlich S, Ulrich M, Piorkowski M, Friedenberger J, et al. Anatomic variables contributing to a higher periprocedural incidence of stroke and TIA in carotid artery stenting: Single center experience of 833 consecutive cases. Catheterization and Cardiovascular Interventions. 2012;**80**(2):321-328

[28] Bazan H, Pradhan S, Mojibian H, Kyriakides T, Dardick A. Increased aortic arch calcification in patients older than 75 years: Implications for carotid artery stenting in elderly patients. Journal of Vascular Surgery. 2007;**46**:841-845

[29] Chiam PT, Roubin GS, Iyer SS, Green RM, Soffer DE, Brennan C, et al. Carotid artery stenting in elderly patients: Importance of case selection. Catheterization and Cardiovascular Interventions. 2008;**72**:318-324

[30] Gribar JJ, Jiddou M, Choksi N, Abbas AE, Bowers T, Kazmierczak C, et al. Carotid stenting in high-risk patients: Early and late outcomes. Journal of Interventional Cardiology. 2011;**24**:247-253

[31] Amarenco P, Cohen A, Tzourio C, Bertrand B, Hommel M, Besson G, et al. Atherosclerotic disease of the aortic arch and the risk of ischemic stroke. The New England Journal of Medicine. 1994;**331**:1474-1479

[32] Davila-Roman VG, Barzailai B, Wareing TH, Murphy SF, Schechtman KB, Kouchoukos NT. Atherosclerosis of the ascending aorta. Prevalence and role as an independent predictor of cerebrovascular events in cardiac patients. Stroke. 1994;**25**:2010-2016

[33] Orlandi G, Fanucchi S, Gallerini S, Sonnoli C, Cosottini M, Puglioli M, et al. Impaired clearance of microemboli and cerebrovascular symptoms during carotid stenting procedures. Archives of Neurology. 2005;**62**:1208-1211

[34] Kar S, Krishnaswamy A, Shishehbor MH, Cam A, Tuzcu EM, Bhatt DL, et al. Safety and efficacy of carotid stenting in individuals with concomitant severe carotid and aortic stenosis. EuroIntervention. 2010;**6**:492-497

[35] Dinculescu V, Ritter AC, dos Santos MP, Mohan RM, Schwarz BA, Lesiuk HJ, et al. Factors determining periprocedural and long-term complications of high risk carotid artery stenting. The Canadian Journal of Neurological Sciences. 2015;**42**(1):48-54

[36] Faggioli G, Ferri M, Gargiulo M, Freyrie A, Fratesi F, Manzoli L, et al. Measurement and impact of proximal and distal tortuosity in carotid stenting procedures. Journal of Vascular Surgery. 2007;**46**(6):1119-1124

[37] Wimmer NJ, Yeh RW, Cutlip DE, Mauri L. Risk prediction for adverse events after carotid artery stenting in higher surgical risk patients. Stroke. 2012;**43**(12):3218-3224

[38] Faggoli G, Ferri M, Rapezzi C, Tonnon C, Manzoli L, Stella A. Atherosclerotic aortic lesions increase the risk of cerebral embolism during carotid stenting in patients with complex aortic arch anatomy. Journal of Vascular Surgery. 2009;**49**:80-85

[39] Dumont TM, Mokin M, Wach MM, Drummond PS, Siddiqui AH, Levy EI, et al. Understanding risk factors for perioperative ischemic events with carotid stenting: Is age over 80 years or is unfavorable arch anatomy to blame. Journal of NeuroInterventional Surgery. 2013;**6**:219-224

[40] Robbs JV, Mulaudzi T, Paruk N, Pillay B, Rajaruthnam P. Carotid intervention: Stent or surgery? A prospective audit. Cardiovascular Journal of Africa. 2009;**20**:336-339

[41] Moore WS. Issues to be addressed and hopefully resolved in the carotid revascularization endarterectomy versus stenting trial 2. Angiology. 2016;**67**:408-410

[42] Derubertis BG, Hynecek RL, Kent KC, Faries PL. Carotid tortuosity in patients with prior cervical radiation: Increased technical challenge during carotid stenting. Vascular and Endovascular Surgery. 2011;**45**:619-626

[43] Fanous AA, Natarajan SK, Jowdy PK, Dumont TM, Mokin M, Yu J, et al. High-risk factors in symptomatic patients undergoing carotid artery stenting with distal protection: Buffalo risk assessment scale (BRASS). Neurosurgery. 2015;**77**:531-542. discussion 542-5

[44] Naggara O, Touzé E, Beyssen B, Trinquart L, Chatellier G, Meder JF, et al. Anatomical and technical factors associated with stroke or death during carotid angioplasty and stenting: Results from the endarterectomy versus angioplasty in patients with symptomatic severe carotid stenosis (EVA-3S) trial and systematic review. Stroke. 2011;**42**:380-388

[45] Stankovic G, Liistro F, Moshiri S, Briguori C, Corvaja N, Gimelli G, et al. Carotid artery stenting in the first 100 consecutive patients: Results and follow up. Heart. 2002;**88**:381-386

[46] Choi HM, Hobson RW, Goldstein J, Chakhtoura E, Lal BK, Haser PB, et al. Technical challenge in a program of carotid artery stenting. Journal of Vascular Surgery. 2004;**40**:746-751

[47] Myouchin K, Takayama K, Taoka T, Nakagawa H, Wada T, Sakamoto M, et al. Carotid Wallstent placement difficulties encountered in carotid artery stenting. Springerplus. 2013;**2**:468

[48] Eskandari MK, Najjar SF, Matsumura JS, Kibbe MR, Morasch MD. Technical limitations of carotid filter embolic protection devices. Annals of Vascular Surgery. 2007;**21**:403-407

[49] Lian X, Liu W, Li M, Lin M, Zhu S, Sun W, et al. Risk factors and complications associated with difficult retrieval ofembolic protection devices in carotid artery stenting. Cardiovascular and Interventional Radiology. 2012;**35**:43-48

[50] Reimers B, Schlüter M, Castriota F, Tübler T, Corvaja N, Cernetti C, et al. Routine use of cerebral protection during carotid artery stenting: Results of a multicenter registry of 753 patients. The American Journal of Medicine. 2004;**116**:217-222

[51] Chong PL, Salhiyyah K, Dodd PDF. The role of carotid endarterectomy in the endovascular era. European Journal of Vascular and Endovascular Surgery. 2005;**29**:597-600

[52] Saw J. Carotid artery stenting for stroke prevention. The Canadian Journal of Cardiology. 2014;**30**:22-34

[53] Saini V, Atchaneeyasakul K, Goswami A, Ambekar S, Ramdas K, Guada L, et al. Safety outcome of carotid artery stenting in long carotid lesion with proximal versus distal embolic protection devices. Neurology. 2017;**88**(16 Supplement):P3.077

[54] Tsutsumi M, Aikawa H, Onizuka M, Iko M, Kodama T, Nii K, et al. Carotid artery stenting for calcified lesions. AJNR. American Journal of Neuroradiology. 2008;**29**(8):1590-1593

[55] Kastrup A, Gröschel K, Schnaudigel S, Nägele T, Schmidt F, Ernemann U. Target lesion ulceration and arch calcification are associated with increased incidence of carotid stenting-associated ischemic lesions in octogenarians. Journal of Vascular Surgery. 2008;**47**(1):88-95

[56] Ricotta JJ, Aburahma A, Ascher E, Eskandari M, Faries P, Lal BK, et al. Updated society for vascular surgery guidelines for management of extracranial carotid disease. Journal of Vascular Surgery. 2011;**54**:e1-e31

[57] Ferguson GG, Eliasziw M, Barr HW, Clagett GP, Barnes RW, Wallace MC, et al. The north American symptomatic carotid endarterectomy trial: Surgical results in 1415 patients. Stroke. 1990;**30**:1751-1758

[58] Inzitari D, Eliasziw M, Gates P, Sharpe BL, Chan RK, Meldrum HE, et al. The causes and risk of stroke in patients with asymptomatic internal-carotid-artery stenosis. North American symptomatic carotid endarterectomy trial collaborators. The New England Journal of Medicine. 2000;**342**:1693-1700

[59] Antoniou GA, Kuhan G, Sfyroeras GS, Georgiadis GS, Antoniou SA, Murray D, et al. Contralateral occlusion of the internal carotid artery increases the risk of patients undergoing carotid endarterectomy. Journal of Vascular Surgery. 2013;**57**:1134-1145

[60] Maatz W, Kohler J, Botsios S, John V, Walterbusch G. Risk of stroke for carotid endarterectomy patients with contralateral occlusion. Annals of Vascular Surgery. 2008;**22**:45-51

[61] Rockman C. Carotid endarterectomy in patients with contralateral carotid occlusion. Seminars in Vascular Surgery. 2004;**17**:224-229

[62] Kretz B, Abello N, Astruc K, Terriat B, Favier C, Bouchot O, et al. Influence of the contralateral carotid artery on carotid surgery outcome. Annals of Vascular Surgery. 2012;**26**:766-774

[63] Rockman CB, Su W, Lamparello PJ, Adelman MA, Jacobowitz GR, Gagne PJ, et al. A reassessment of carotid endarterectomy in the face of contralateral carotid occlusion: Surgical results in symptomatic and asymptomatic patients. Journal of Vascular Surgery. 2002;**36**:668-673

[64] Mackey WC, O'Donnell TF Jr, Callow AD. Carotid endarterectomy contralateral to an occluded carotid artery: Perioperative risk and late results. Journal of Vascular Surgery. 1990;**11**:778-783

[65] Dalainas I, Nano G, Bianchi P, Casana R, Malacrida G, Tealdi DG. Carotid endarterectomy in patients with contralateral carotid artery occlusion. Annals of Vascular Surgery. 2007;**21**:16-22

[66] Grego F, Antonello M, Lepidi S, Zaramella M, Galzignan E, Menegolo M, et al. Is contralateral carotid artery occlusion a risk factor for carotid endarterectomy? Annals of Vascular Surgery. 2005;**19**:882-889

[67] Pulli R, Dorigo W, Barbanti E, Azas L, Russo D, Matticari S, et al. Carotid endarterectomy with contralateral carotid artery occlusion: Is this a higher risk subgroup? European Journal of Vascular and Endovascular Surgery. 2002;**24**:63-68

[68] Halm EA, Tuhrim S, Wang JJ, Rockman C, Riles TS, Chassin MR. Risk factors for perioperative death and stroke after carotid endarterectomy: Results of the New York carotid artery surgery study. Stroke. 2009;**40**:221-229

[69] Yang SS, Kim YW, Kim DI, Kim KH, Jeon P, Kim GM, et al. Impact of contralateral carotid or vertebral artery occlusion in patients undergoing carotid endarterectomy or carotid artery stenting. Journal of Vascular Surgery. 2014;**59**(3):749-755

[70] Lee JH, Choi CG, Kim DK, Kim GE, Lee HK, Suh DC. Relationship between circle of Willis morphology on 3D time-of-flight MR angiograms and transient ischemia during vascular clamping of the internal carotid artery during carotid endarterectomy. AJNR. American Journal of Neuroradiology. 2004;**25**:558-564

[71] Sabeti S, Schillinger M, Mlekusch W, Nachtmann T, Lang W, Ahmadi R, et al. Contralateral high-grade carotid artery stenosis or occlusion is not associated with increased risk for poor neurologic outcome after elective carotid stent placement. Radiology. 2004; **230**:70-76

[72] Keldahl ML, Park MS, Garcia-Toca M, Wang CH, Kibbe MR, Rodriguez HE, et al. Does a contralateral carotid occlusion adversely impact carotid artery stenting outcomes? Annals of Vascular Surgery. 2012;**26**:40-45

[73] Lago A, Parkhutik V, Tembl JI, Aparici F, Mainar E, Alcala C, et al. Long-term outcome in patients with carotid artery stenting and contralateral carotid occlusion: A single neurovascular center prospective analysis. Neuroradiology. 2012;**54**:965-972

[74] Mercado N, Cohen DJ, Spertus JA, Chan PS, House J, Kennedy K, et al. Carotid artery stenting of a contralateral occlusion and in-hospital outcomes: Results from the CARE (carotid artery revascularization and endarterectomy) registry. JACC. Cardiovascular Interventions. 2013;**6**:59-64

[75] Nicolau C, Gilabert R, Garcia A, Blasco J, Chamorro A, Bru C. Effect of internal carotid artery occlusion on vertebral artery blood flow: A duplex ultrasonographic evaluation. Journal of Ultrasound in Medicine. 2001;**20**:105-111

[76] Hoffmann A, Dinkel M, Schweiger H, Lang W. The influence of the state of the vertebral arteries on the peri- and postoperative risk in carotid surgery. European Journal of Vascular and Endovascular Surgery. 1998;**16**:329-333

[77] Koren-Morag N, Goldbourt U, Tanne D. Renal dysfunction and risk of ischemic stroke or TIA in patients with cardiovascular disease. Neurology. 2006;**67**:224-228

[78] Maeda N, Sawayama Y, Tatsukawa M, et al. Carotid artery lesions and atherosclerotic risk factors in Japanese hemodialysis patients. Atherosclerosis. 2003;**169**:183-192

[79] Fleisher LA, Beckman JA, Brown KA, et al. ACC/AHA 2007 guidelines on perioperative cardiovascular evaluation and care for noncardiac surgery: A report of the American College of Cardiology/American Heart Association task force on practice guidelines (writing committee to revise the 2002 guideline). Circulation. 2007;**116**:e418-e499

[80] AbuRahma AF, Srivastava M, Chong B, Dean LS, Stone PA, Koszewski A. Impact of chronic renal insufficiency using serum creatinine vs glomerular filtration rate on perioperative clinical outcomes of carotid endarterectomy. Journal of the American College of Surgeons. 2013;**216**:525-532

[81] Tarakji A, McConaughy A, Nicholas GG. The risk of carotid endarterectomy in patients with chronic renal insufficiency. Current Surgery. 2006;**63**:326-329

[82] Rigdon EE, Monajjem N, Rhodes RS. Is carotid endarterectomy justified in patients with severe chronic renal insufficiency? Annals of Vascular Surgery. 1997;**11**:115-119

[83] Donahue M, Visconti G, Focaccio A, Selvetella L, Baldassarre M, Viviani Anselmi C, et al. Acute kidney injury in patients with chronic kidney disease undergoing internal carotid artery stent implantation. JACC. Cardiovascular Interventions. 2015;**8**(11):1506-1514

[84] Saw J, Gurm HS, Fathi RB, et al. Effect of chronic kidney disease on outcomes after carotid artery stenting. The American Journal of Cardiology. 2004;**94**:1093-1096

[85] Gruberg L, Jeremias A, Rundback JH, et al. Impact of glomerular filtration rate on clinical outcomes following carotid artery revascularization in 11,832 patients from the care registry(R). Catheterization and Cardiovascular Interventions. 2014;**84**:246-254

[86] Adil MM, Saeed F, Chaudhary SA, Malik A, Qureshi AI. Comparative outcomes of carotid artery stent placement and carotid endarterectomy in patients with chronic kidney disease and end-stage renal disease. Journal of Stroke and Cerebrovascular Diseases. 2016;**25**(7):1721-1727

Chapter 3

Diagnostic Imaging of Carotid Artery

Lachezar Manchev

Additional information is available at the end of the chapter

http://dx.doi.org/10.5772/intechopen.79762

Abstract

In the study of carotid arteries, the different imaging techniques allow to analyze various diseases like stenoses, aneurysms, thromboses, dissections, diseases caused by atherosclerotic plaques or congenital abnormalities. The diagnostic modalities that are used to image the carotid artery diseases are digital subtraction angiography (DSA), duplex ultrasound (DUS), computed tomography angiography (CTA), and magnetic resonance angiography (MRA). The goal of the diagnostic imaging is to provide screening and to detect diseases at its earliest and most treatable stage. As initial screening study, the radiologists recommend DUS. It is a safe and painless way to produce pictures of the inside of the body using sound waves. It assesses blood flow in the carotid arteries, measures the speed of the blood flow, and estimates the diameter of a blood vessel and degree of obstruction. Digital subtraction angiography (DSA) has assumed a major role in the evaluation of occlusive cerebrovascular disease. While digital subtraction angiography (DSA) is still considered the gold standard, it has increasingly been replaced by computed tomography angiography (CTA) or magnetic resonance angiography (MRA) during the last years. Modern imaging studies like CTA and MRI allow to obtain three-dimensional reconstruction of anatomic structures and pathological abnormalities. Computed tomography angiography (CTA) of carotid arteries is a standardized procedure with excellent image quality but related with high radiation exposure. The rapid technical evolution in hardware and software allows even smaller imaging centers to perform high-quality vessel imaging. During the last decade, CTA came up with substantial progress in terms of accuracy in stenosis and aneurysm detection. Magnetic resonance angiography (MRA) is increasingly used as a noninvasive method to assess carotid arteries. Diseases like carotid artery dissections could be detected by using MRA or CTA.

Keywords: carotid artery, Doppler ultrasound, digital subtraction angiography, computed tomography angiography, magnetic resonance angiography

1. Introduction

In general, diagnostic imaging studies of the carotid artery diseases are divided into two large groups: noninvasive in which there is no contact with the patient's bloodstream and invasive in which such a contact exists.

2. Noninvasive methods

2.1. Doppler ultrasound (DUS)

Doppler ultrasound is a nontraumatic method that allows getting information about the linear and volumetric blood flow velocity in the carotid, vertebral, and other arteries; it is used to determine the degree of vessel stenosis and obturations and to outline the pathways of collateral circulation. The capabilities of Doppler ultrasound to determine the condition of carotid and vertebral arteries are verified by brain angiography, the coincidences reaching a high percentage. Doppler ultrasound is based on the Doppler effect, which refers to the change of sound, ultrasound, and light wave frequencies when they are reflected by a moving object. This phenomenon is used in the Doppler ultrasound exam, where erythrocytes and other forms of blood elements in the blood vessels are the moving objects.

2.2. Ultrasound methods for cerebral artery examination

2.2.1. Ultrasound scan

Ultrasound scanning (echography, B-mode) is a two-dimensional imaging in one plane, based on the reflection and diffusion of ultrasound rays from different density tissues. The ultrasound amplitude of the reflected signal is displayed on the screen as a point of varying grayscale intensity—white and black. Scanning is performed by a great number of parallel ultrasound rays, which pass through the scanned object with a frequency of 10–60 pulsations per second. Different frequency instant images of the scanned object appear during these ultrasound pulsations of reflected rays. Thus, vessels can be seen in motion. This real-time pulse scanning method is used in modern equipment. In that way, anatomical structures can be displayed on a two-dimensional plane in ultrasound scanning [1–7].

2.2.2. Continuous-wave Doppler ultrasound

Continuous-wave Doppler ultrasound is the most common modern ultrasound method for examining extracranial cerebral arteries, peripheral arteries, and veins. The diagnostic frequency of the ultrasound emission is from 2 to 20 MHz. Deeper vessels are examined with transducers for a lower frequency of the ultrasound emission [8, 9].

2.2.3. Spectral analysis of the Doppler signal

The objectivization of Doppler ultrasound is performed through spectral quantitative analysis of its frequency and amplitude characteristics. Frequency or velocity analysis of Doppler ultrasound, which is an expression of the blood flow velocity, is most widely used in all Doppler ultrasound exams. The Doppler velocity curve gives an approximate idea about the average velocity of the blood flow, passing through the artery cross section. In case of accelerated or turbulent blood flow due to artery stenosis, the velocity of a part of the erythrocytes changes dramatically and some of them receive a retrograde flow due to vortex formation. These changes may not significantly affect blood flow average velocity and velocity curve, but they change the Doppler frequency spectrum significantly [10].

The amplitude or power spectrum shows the quantitative distribution of the power of movement of all blood components over a certain short interval of time in the cardiac cycle. In stenosis, the frequency or velocity increases, but the power of blood flow decreases due to turbulence, and therefore, the increase and especially the drop in amplitude is slow and the amplitude peak is low and shifted to low frequencies. Spectral width is an important indicator of amplitude analysis as it reflects the frequency, respectively the velocity, corresponding to 70% of the maximum blood flow power. This indicator makes it possible to assess the degree of damage to laminar blood flow in the presence of turbulence.

2.2.4. *Transcranial Doppler ultrasound (TCD)*

This method makes it possible to simultaneously visualize the intensity and direction of the blood flow at different depths in the intracranial space. It provides information on the condition of the arteries emerging from the Circle of Willis. With this methodology, it is possible to select the most optimal Doppler signal from one or more different depths. This is convenient for monitoring the path of microembolic signals that are presented as high-amplitude signals through arterial blood flow. Transcranial Doppler sonography allows the monitoring of microemboli that emerge from the middle cerebral artery (MCA), proximal to stenosis, and chronic stenosis of the said artery. Fifty-eight patients with chronic stenosis of the MCA were examined. Twenty-three of them (29.5%) have low-grade stenosis, 18 (23%) had moderate-grade stenosis, while 37 (47.5%) were diagnosed with severe stenoses. Thirty-seven of the stenoses were symptomatic, and 41 were with asymptomatic carotid stenosis (ACS). Two ischemic strokes and seven transient ischemic attacks (TIAs) were observed during the follow-up. Twenty-four patients were treated with anticoagulants and 28 received aspirin. Microembolic signals were found in symptomatic and asymptomatic stenoses regardless of the medication received. These results indicate that chronic middle artery stenoses do not represent a significant source of emboli [11]. Transcranial Doppler sonography also allows for the monitoring of intracranial blood vessels in patients who had undergone thrombolysis [12] and also for the emergency diagnosis of ischemic stroke following head trauma [13].

2.2.5. *Extracranial Doppler ultrasound imaging*

The method makes it possible to visualize extracranial brain vessels using the Doppler effect. Doppler sonography shows Doppler spectral analysis, which includes all velocities of the examined blood flow segment and an analog Doppler curve representing the mean velocity of the examined bloodstream segment.

2.2.6. Color-coded duplex Doppler ultrasound imaging

This method makes it possible to simultaneously analyze the blood flow of the studied artery in several separate blood volumes. A two-dimensional image of the velocity of all blood volumes and blood flow direction is obtained in a plane, the images being encoded in different colors. The resulting images are in real time [14, 15].

2.2.7. Duplex scanning

It is a combination of echography, a real-time B-scanner, and a single-channel pulsed Doppler ultrasound system. In this way, the blood flow in the studied artery can be determined, as well as its speed and direction. The ultrasound determines the diameter of the vessel and the angle at which the ultrasound pulsating waves enter the longitudinal axis of the artery under study. Thus, these methods combine and complement each other. The method is used to examine the extracranial parts of the carotid arteries, the initial parts of the vertebral and subclavian arteries [16].

2.2.8. Spectral analysis of the Doppler signal in cerebral artery stenosis

An increase in the blood flow velocity is observed with acceleration of the systolic and diastolic part of the spectral form and the Doppler curve in the area above the stenosis. The laminar nature of the bloodstream is distorted, it becomes deformed and turbulent. After the stenosis, there is a slowing of blood flow and a turbulence increase [17].

2.2.9. Ultrasound diagnosis of atheromatous plaques

The method is important for clinical diagnosis because atherosclerotic plaques narrow the lumen of the blood vessel on the one hand and, on the other hand, are a source of emboli to the cerebral vessels.

The most informative method for the detection of atherosclerotic plaques, originating from the vascular wall and various calcifications, is echography (B-mode). These plaques are often found in the arterial bifurcations and the end portions of the internal carotid artery [17].

3. Angiographic methods

3.1. Digital subtraction angiography

In the angiographic method, the vascular system of the brain is examined following the introduction of a contrast agent into the arteries. According to the type of arteries examined, we distinguish between carotid and vertebral angiography.

Diagnostic possibilities of digital subtraction angiography (DSA) were investigated in the diagnosis of cerebrovascular disease. A retrospective analysis was performed in 65 patients with various forms of cerebrovascular disease, taking into account the clinical characteristics and the risks accompanying them. In 75.4% of the patients, DSA found changes, with 85.5% having ischemic disorders of the cerebral circulation. The main diseases that led to the development of cerebrovascular disease were cerebral artery stenosis or atherosclerotic occlusions mainly in the extracranial vessels. Intraventricular hemorrhage was detected in four patients, and five patients had subarachnoid hemorrhage. Still DSA continues to be a gold standard in the diagnostics of the cerebrovascular disease.

3.2. Computed tomography angiography

Computed tomography angiography is an accurate means of determining intracranial occlusion in patients within the first 6 h of the onset of the cerebrovascular accident.

Computed tomography 3D-CT angiography of cerebral vessels is a technique that is particularly useful in the diagnosis of brain lesions and cerebrovascular disease. However, it does not provide information on the dynamics of blood flow changes. Therefore, a new technique has been developed—dynamic (D3D-CTA) angiography, which gives a 3D image of the vessels and allows assessment of hemodynamics and cerebral perfusion. Twelve patients were examined with CTA D3D (seven with brain tumors, four with arteriovenous malformations, and one with occlusion of the inner carotid artery). For all patients, information on changes in vascular structures, hemodynamics, and cerebral perfusion status was provided. Despite the relatively high risks, related to exposure to radiation, and limited scanning range, this technique is useful in the diagnosis of patients with cerebrovascular disease and brain tumors [18–21].

3.3. 3D-CT arteriography and 3D-CT venography

Although 3D-CT angiography provides valuable anatomical information regarding the lesion and the adjacent vascular and bone structures, it cannot show lesions of the arteries and veins individually. 3D-CT venography allows for a more detailed study of vascular anatomy and allows improvement of the diagnosis and potentially safe surgical approach [20].

3.4. Magnetic resonance angiography (MRA)

It is a method of obtaining blood vessel images by using magnetic resonance. This method allows the assessment of the anatomical and functional characteristics of the bloodstream. Under the influence of a strong magnetic field, rotation of the hydrogen nuclei protons occurs and they change their location, positioning themselves along the magnetic field axis. The effects of the magnetic field and the radiofrequency emission of the protons are not constant and have no certain force, frequency, and time; after the radio frequency influence, the protons again return to the starting position, i.e., T1 and T2. The effects of the magnetic field and the radio frequency impulse of the hydrogen nuclei protons force them to rotate in relatively new axes over a very short period of time, which is accompanied by the emission and absorption of energy and the formation of their own magnetic field. The registration of these energy changes is the basis of the MRI image. The magnetic resonance angiography method allows obtaining images of the vessels without the use of any contrasting agents, but, in order to achieve a clearer picture, various contrast agents based on gadolinium can be used. The method finds less application for evaluation of carotid stenoses [22, 23].

IEFNS set up a working group with the aim of developing basic guidelines for the treatment and prevention of stroke patients in line with local and national requirements of neurologists from Europe. Due to increased population aging across Europe and socioeconomic and health issues, the opinion that the incidence and severity of ischemic strokes will increase in many countries over the next decades was formed. In addition, acute stroke mortality rate varies considerably across European countries, being the highest in many East European countries and considerably lower in West European countries. It was emphasized that the viability of ischemic brain tissue can be extended to 18 or even 24 h, experimental studies showing that the earlier intervention leads to a more favorable outcome. Thrombolysis is recommended to be used within a therapeutic window of up to 3 h after stroke, and it is currently being investigated whether it will be effective until the sixth hour. Neuroprotective agents are recommended up to 12 h from the vascular accident. The factors, delaying the onset of treatment due to later referral to a hospital, can be overcome if neurologists participate in special educational programs to improve initial diagnosis and manage emergency situations.

There is an urgent need for a variety of diagnostic methods: computed tomography, Doppler sonography, electrocardiography, echocardiography, and laboratory tests, including coagulation status testing. Cardiac monitoring, blood pressure, blood gases, and body temperature monitoring are essential. If necessary, angiography, NMR, and EEG monitoring should be performed. After alleviation of the acute stroke, it is advisable to refer the patient to a rehabilitation unit.

A European guideline for the diagnosis of acute strokes was established. It emphasizes the need for neuroimaging techniques in the assessment of acute stroke, one of the leading causes of death and lasting neurological disabilities in developed countries. A comprehensive review of the literature, published in English for the period 1965–2005, was conducted and a set of methods for diagnosing stroke was created. Native CT of the brain is the first method of choice in diagnosis. Magnetic resonance tomography is a more sensitive computed tomography method and is particularly useful in the assessment of ischemic areas as well as in the diagnosis of acute and chronic intracerebral hemorrhages. Perfusion computed tomography and magnetic resonance angiography (MRA) are also very useful. MRT and MRA are the recommended techniques for the screening of brain aneurysms and for the diagnosis of cerebral venous thrombosis and arterial dissection. For noninvasive extra- and intracranial vessels study, extracranial and transcranial Doppler sonography are very useful. The transcranial Doppler sonography examination is very useful for monitoring arterial reperfusion after thrombolysis, for diagnosing intracranial stenosis and the presence of shunts, and for monitoring vasospasm after subarachnoid hemorrhage. Currently, single-photon emission computed tomography (SPECT) and positron emission tomography (PET) have a more limited role in acute cerebral strokes assessment [24].

A number of other scientific publications emphasize the role of neuroimaging techniques in brain stroke patients [24–27].

4. Combination of diagnostic imaging studies for carotid artery diseases

4.1. Transcranial Doppler sonography, CT angiography, digital subtraction angiography, and MR angiography

In modern emergency stroke therapy, many patients may temporarily improve, especially after thrombolysis, and worsen again to the original neurological deficit. Although mechanisms of such deterioration (DFI) may include development of brain edema, reperfusion hemorrhage, or other secondary factors such as cardiopulmonary decompensation, most DFIs are due to indefinite processes. Urgent sonographic assessment of patients with acute neurological deficits and DFI is not well characterized. The aim of the study was to evaluate the incidence and characteristics of vascular lesions in determining the acute spontaneous development of deficits and their potential links with subsequent DFI. Patients with focal neurologic deficit associated with cerebral ischemia, which was evaluated with a total NIH stroke score < 4 within 6 h of onset of symptoms, were prospectively studied.

Transcranial Doppler sonography (TCD) was routinely used and, when necessary, subsequent digital subtraction angiography (DSA), CT angiography (CTA), or MR angiography (MRA) was used. Vascular images were interpreted by a neurologist and a neuroradiologist for the presence of occlusions of large arterial vessels, stenoses, etc. Occlusions of large vessels were evaluated as atherosclerotic, in which Doppler sonography or angiography showed narrowing or occlusion of extra- and intracranial arteries greater than 50%. Stroke cases in which the potential source of emboli had been found were classified as embolic. In other cases, arterial dissection or coagulopathy was accepted as the cause of the stroke, and in some cases, the mechanism remained undetermined. Fifty patients with an average age of 61 + 14 years were studied, the women being 50%. The patients' symptoms had occurred after 165 + 96 min. Transcranial Doppler sonography was performed in all patients, and subsequent angiographic studies (DSA 10%, CTA 4%, MRA 44%) were performed in 68%. In general, large artery occlusions during TCD exam were found in 16% of patients, stenosis was found in 18%, 54% had normal studies, and the study could not be performed in 10%. DFI was observed in 16% of patients, TCD and angiography showed occlusion data in 62%, 22% had stenosis, and 4% of the vascular exams had normal results. DFI occurred in 31% of patients with atherosclerosis in a large arterial vessel, 23% had cardiac embolism, and 9% had small vessels damaged. In conclusion, it is emphasized that DFIs are strongly associated with the presence of occlusion or narrowing of a large arterial vessel of atherosclerotic or embolic origin. The reliability of emergency TCD or angiography in the early diagnosis of vascular lesions is very high. This makes it possible to assess the condition of the patients and to determine the therapeutic strategy [4, 28, 29].

A 3D visualization method was established for the entire vascular system, which includes carotid and vertebral arteries. Spiral CT angiography (SCTA) was used, providing a precise, qualitative, and quantitative assessment of anatomical abnormalities, including the detection of additional lesions and an assessment of the degree of stenosis. Fifteen patients with pathological abnormalities of the arterial vascular system, detected by color-coded duplex ultrasound, were examined using digital subtraction angiography (IA-DSA) and SCTA. The results obtained from 3D SCTA showed a high correlation with those of IA-DSA and SCTA [30].

Severe intracranial artery stenosis is the main cause of acute ischemic stroke. Although the warning symptoms for such stenosis are rarely found, cerebral transient ischemic attacks and ischemic stroke require active and effective diagnosis and treatment. The study described the main diagnostic methods for the diagnosis of arterial stenosis. Digital subtraction angiography makes it possible to trace the entire vascular system by conducting dynamic observations through the introduction of contrast agent. Magnetic resonance angiography also provides information but cannot properly show changes in small blood vessels. Transcranial Doppler sonography makes it possible for the changes in large intracranial vessels, the blood flow velocity, etc., to be detected by noninvasive technique. In computed tomography angiography, performed with intravenous contrasting of iodine contrast media, the vessels of Circle of Willis can be examined.

Medical professionals should use different imaging techniques to evaluate patients with stroke. The main diagnostic methods are used in these cases. Computer tomography allows a series of brain slices to be made, excluding hemorrhage or brain tumor. Abnormal findings can usually be observed during a computed tomography scan from 6 to 8 h after the onset of stroke. Another diagnostic method is magnetic resonance tomography. Its advantage is that it can show brain edema a few hours after the stroke and is better than computed tomography in detecting small cerebral infarctions. Doppler sonography is a noninvasive method for investigating extra- and intracranial vessels. Other methods, used in acute stroke diagnosis, are magnetic resonance and conventional angiography, which is performed under stricter indications [11].

The diagnostic merits of Doppler imaging, CT angiography, and digital subtraction angiography (DSA) for diagnosing carotid stenosis have been compared. DSA is considered a "gold standard" for confirming severe stenoses (70–99%) of internal carotid arteries; yet it is associated with a risk of complications. The aim of the study was to evaluate the accuracy of Doppler sonography, computed tomographic angiography, and their combined use for the detection and quantification of severe carotid stenosis as compared to DSA. 29 patients were included in the study and their results were compared. The results showed that DUS in combination with STA can be used for relatively reliable diagnosis of severe stenoses of the internal carotid artery. Thus, invasive digital subtraction angiography can be avoided in a significant number of patients [31].

Computed tomography angiography (CTA) is a relatively new and minimally invasive method of visualizing the intracranial and extracranial blood vessels. The diagnostic capabilities of the CTA and the gold standard of arterial imaging (DSA) were compared. A total of 40 patients (80 carotid arteries), examined with STA, DUS, and DSA, were prospectively studied. Patients, selected for inclusion, had symptoms of cerebral transient ischemic attacks or stroke. The degree of stenosis and atheromatous changes were studied by the three methods. The results showed that STA had significant correlations with DSA, while the correlation with DUS was less obvious. STA showed good possibilities for detecting light carotid stenoses (0–29%) and arterial occlusions. Stenosis detection of more than 50% was achieved with DSA, while CTA showed a sensitivity of about 50%. In addition, CTA showed quite good correlations with DSA in detecting lesion atheromatous plaques in carotid stenosis. In conclusion, CTA shows very good capabilities for detection of carotid artery occlusions or stenosis up to 50% but is not able to reliably distinguish the differences between moderate (50–69%) and severe (70–99%) stenoses, which is important in determining the methods for the treatment of carotid stenosis [18].

Invasive diagnosing imaging of cervical and intracranial vessels, done with CTA, MRA, and DUS, has been studied in other clinical trials as well [32].

4.2. Transcranial Doppler ultrasound, MR angiography, and digital subtraction angiography

Single-slice CT angiography (CTA) is an established method for imaging the vascular system of the brain (CVS), but it suffers from technical limitations for the visualization of long vascular segments such as intra- and extracranial vessels. The comparatively recently created multislice (MS) technology allows high-quality angiographic images due to increased scanning speeds and improved spatial resolution. The study was aimed at assessing the suitability of multislice CTA (MS-CTA) when examining the vascular system of patients with acute symptoms of arterial and venous occlusion. In 41 patients with a clinical suspicion of acute cerebral ischemia (29 in the hemisphere and 12 in the vertebrobasilar system), as well as in 4 patients with suspicion of cerebral venous thrombosis, MS-CTA was administered. Additionally, Doppler sonography was performed in 34 patients, magnetic resonance angiography in 5 patients, and digital subtraction angiography in 6 patients. All findings for extra- and intracranial blood vessel stenoses were correlated with clinical outcomes. The study showed that MS-CTA is a promising diagnostic tool for rapid and overall assessment of arterial and venous vessels in patients with clinical signs of acute cerebrovascular disease [33, 34].

Transcranial Doppler sonography (TCD) may localize arterial occlusion in patients with stroke. About 190 patients with, or without, proximal extra- and intracranial occlusions were examined by TCD. The obtained data were compared with those from DSA and MRA. Angiographic examination showed occlusion in 48 patients. The TCD showed Doppler signals unusual for the middle cerebral artery in 66.7%; reverse blood flow through the ophthalmic arteries in 70.6%; and blood flow through the anterior communicating artery in 78.6% and through the posterior communicating artery in 71.4%. The study showed that transcranial Doppler sonography data for large artery occlusions can be used to extend complex diagnosis and improve prognostic value for noninvasive screening in stroke patients [35].

For a very long time, medical professionals believed that arteriography is a mandatory method for diagnosing the dissection of the internal carotid artery. With the introduction of transcranial Doppler sonography and magnetic resonance angiography, it is no longer the case. Thirteen patients with dissection of the internal carotid artery were diagnosed by extra- and transcranial Doppler sonography, computed tomography, and magnetic resonance tomography. Digital subtraction angiography, as a "gold standard," confirmed the diagnosis in all cases. Thus, noninvasive techniques can be sufficiently informative in such patients [36].

The diagnostic capabilities of digital intra-arterial angiography and transcranial Doppler sonography were compared in 48 patients with acute cerebral ischemia in the carotid artery basin on the fourth hour after onset of symptoms. Data from the TCD exam showed correlation with angiographic examination.

The clinical manifestations of vascular hypoplasia were studied in 205 children aged 3–14 years. About 21% of them had transient ischemic attacks (TIAs), and 17% had cerebral infarction; focal or generalized epileptic seizures were found in 56.1%, while 4.9% had migraine headache. Cerebral arterial hypoplasia was diagnosed with angiography, MR angiography, and transcranial Doppler sonography [37].

Acute occlusion of the basilar artery is a common condition, but differential diagnosis is not always easy for patients with acute onset, change in consciousness, and progressive dysfunction of the brainstem. Intra-arterial thrombolytic therapy is a potential life-saving procedure in certain cases of acute occlusion of the basilar artery. Therefore, it is necessary to have reliable and widely available methods for assessing the patency of the basilar artery. Traditionally, digital subtraction angiography has been used for diagnosis in suspected cases of acute occlusion of the basilar artery. However, DSA is a laborious, costly, and invasive method that requires patient cooperation or general anesthesia. Extra- and intracranial Doppler sonography was used to diagnose clinical suspicion of acute occlusion of the basilar artery. Unfortunately, due to DUS technical limitations, especially for the study of distal portions of the vertebral artery, ultrasound diagnosis may be inadequate.

Magnetic resonance angiography has not been used so far in large groups of patients for the examination of the basilar artery occlusion. Difficulties can be explained with the specific patients' condition—disturbed consciousness and intubation in patients with acute cerebral ischemia.

Spiral CT angiography (CTA) is a relatively new instrumental method for noninvasive vascular diagnosis in cases of acute cerebral ischemia. A prospective study was conducted with 19 patients of an average age of 58 + 11 years with clinical suspicion of acute vertebral artery occlusion. Criteria for inclusion of the patients were the clinical manifestations of sudden worsening of consciousness, dizziness, diplopia, dysarthria, oculomotor nerve lesions, and lesions of other cranial nerves or bilateral symptoms. Three patients were in coma. The diagnostic capabilities of CTA, DUS, and DSA, used for these patients, were compared. CTA revealed a complete occlusion of the basilar artery in nine patients and an incomplete occlusion in two of them. Due to severe vertebral artery calcification, one patient could not be examined. Doppler sonography was performed in 7 of 19 patients, with clear evidence of vertebral artery occlusion in 3 of them. In the remaining patients, the data were uncertain and two were false-negative, which was proved by CTA and DSA exams. In addition, CTA provided information on the exact place of basilar artery occlusion. These data allowed for intra-arterial thrombolysis to be used in five patients. In conclusion, CTA was more informative than DUS in assessing the patency of the basilar artery in patients with acute ischemia, especially in the distal artery occlusion. The study emphasizes the advantages of the combination of methods, used for the diagnosis of basilar artery occlusion [38].

The role of CTA, MR angiography, DUS, and DSA for the quantification of atherosclerotic stenosis of the carotid artery was studied in 25 patients. The degree of stenosis was measured according to North American Symptomatic Carotid Endarterectomy Criteria: complete occlusion (100%), severe (70–99%), moderate (30–69%), and mild (0–29%). Degree of stenosis, measured by CTA, MRA, and DUS (Doppler ultrasound), was compared to the DSA results, used as the "gold standard." Ninety-seven percent of the results obtained from MRA were equivalent to DSA and 3% did not match; 96% of CTA data were DSA equivalents, with 4% not matched; 77% of the results of Doppler sonography were equivalent to DSA, and 23% had a mismatch. In conclusion, it is emphasized that CTA and MRA are equally accurate methods for quantification of the degree of stenosis in carotid bifurcation [39].

In 178 patients with cerebrovascular disease, studies were conducted to compare whether invasive CT angiography was an alternative to digital subtraction angiography and noninvasive Doppler sonography. CTA reported nine cases of significant stenosis, which were not thoroughly assessed by the DSA, and in two cases, it did not show any results. In addition, vascular wall calcifications were more easily evaluated by CTA [40].

4.3. Transcranial Doppler ultrasound and CT angiography

Atherosclerotic diseases of the middle cerebral artery (MCA) are often met with Asian population. This abnormality can be diagnosed by noninvasive methods such as transcranial Doppler ultrasound (TCD) and CT angiography (CT). The diagnostic capabilities of these two methods were compared in 70 patients with suspicion of atherothrombotic occlusion of the middle cerebral artery. The study excluded cases of cardiac embolism, significant carotid stenosis, or classical lacunar syndrome. Transcranial Doppler ultrasound was performed within 2 days of hospitalizing the patients; it was followed by STA within 7 days of stroke. CTA showed stenoses of MSA exceeding 50% in 57 patients (81%), whereas only 29 patients (41%) had TCD visualized abnormalities. TCD results correlate well with those of CTA in all patients with proximal stenosis of the M1 segment. In contrast, transcranial Doppler sonography visualizes accurately distal M1 or M2 injuries only in 24% of patients. In this population, CTA showed better abilities than TCD in the diagnosis of thrombosis of MCA. Transcranial Doppler sonography should not be used as a basic method for the detection of MCA stenoses [41].

A pilot study of the diagnostic capabilities of CTA and TCD in the diagnosis of intracranial occlusion of intracerebral arteries was performed. Ten patients with acute ischemic stroke as a result of stenosis or MCA occlusion were studied. Seven stenoses and five occlusions of MCA were found. CTA confirmed all TCD results except for one patient with MCA occlusion, who had multiple embolisms. The results showed that CTA is an easily performed and useful method in the diagnosis of MCA occlusion [42]. A number of other studies have shown the high diagnostic value of TCD and CT angiography in basilar artery stenosis and occlusions [38].

Transcranial color-coded duplex sonography (TCCD), magnetic resonance angiography (MRA), and computed tomography angiography (CT) are relatively new noninvasive or minimally invasive techniques to study intracranial circulation. TCCD makes it possible to improve the accuracy and reliability of data supplied by conventional transcranial Doppler imaging. The main limitation of transcranial color-coded duplex sonography is related to the ultrasound windows that make it difficult to insonate the basilar arteries, especially in their proximal part, and has a lower resolution. MRA provides good morphological information on the condition of the cerebral vessels. CTA is a sensitive method for detecting occlusive changes in the large intracranial arteries. Transcranial color-coded duplex sonography and magnetic resonance angiography, used in combination or alone, can eliminate the need for digital subtraction angiography in most cases of occlusive cerebrovascular disease. Digital subtraction angiography can be used in cases where noninvasive techniques do not provide sufficient information, or for the diagnosis of brain aneurysms and arteriovenous malformations. The role of CTA for the detection of aneurysms by contrast agent injection is well established, whereas in cases of other lesions, the method does not always produce clear results [10].

Patients with acute ischemic stroke, having occurred with intracranial arterial obstructions, are with poor prognosis and a high probability of death up to 24 h. The diagnostic accuracy of Doppler ultrasound (PMD-TCD) and CT angiography is assessed as a standard in the diagnosis of intracranial artery occlusion in patients with ischemic stroke within 24 h. A total of 100 patients were studied. PMD-TCD showed intracranial occlusion in 34 patients, while the STA showed the same result in 33 patients. Six false-positive and four false-negative diagnoses were found by PMD-TCD. This methodology showed a high coincidence with CT angiography in the diagnosis of occlusion of arterial vessels in patients with acute ischemic stroke, especially in the middle cerebral artery basin [43].

4.4. CT angiography and digital subtraction angiography

A study was conducted to determine whether spiral CT angiography allows accurate quantitative assessment of anatomical abnormalities, including the detection of additional lesions, determining plaque morphology, and assessment of carotid artery stenosis. The diagnostic capabilities of spiral CT angiography and digital subtraction angiography were compared in 92 cases of carotid artery stenosis. The degree of stenosis was determined according to the North American Symptomatic Carotid Endarterectomy Trial (NASCET). All stenoses were diagnosed using CT angiography. It showed coincidence with digital subtraction angiography in 59% of the cases with mild stenosis, in 82% of the cases with moderate stenosis, and in 90% of those with severe stenosis. Calcified plaques were easily detected by spiral CT angiography, but discovery of lesion plaques was difficult. The study showed that spiral CT angiography gives enough information for carotid stenoses greater than 30% and for calcified plaque detection but is not sufficiently informative for detecting lesions [44].

Carotid artery examination is important for the evaluation of patients with ischemic stroke and cerebral transient ischemic accidents. CT angiography (CTA) of the head and neck is an easily accessible method that can be part of the routine imaging diagnosis in patients with stroke. In a large academic center, for the period 2000–2002, CTA and DSA examinations of the cervical part of the carotid artery were performed in 81 patients according to the NASCET criteria. For stenoses over 70%, the coincidence of both methods was 96%. The study showed that CTA is an excellent screening test for stenosis of the internal carotid artery [45].

Intravenous recombinant tissue plasminogen activator (TPA) has been shown to be effective in the treatment of acute ischemic stroke within the first 3 h of onset, but unfortunately the occlusion of the vessel may not always be well documented in due time. Digital subtraction angiography, performed within several hours, is a method of quickly and reliably validating the intracranial occlusion of the vessel. CT angiography is also potentially useful for this purpose, as it shows significant coincidence with DSA. About 54 patients with acute stroke were examined using the two methodologies. CTA has shown coincidence with DSA regarding occlusions in 86% of the cases [7].

The possibilities of multidetector CTA as compared to DSA were studied in 35 patients (70 carotid arteries). The degree of stenosis was calculated according to NASCET. CTA was somewhat inaccurate for measuring the absolute minimum diameter in high-grade stenoses, while in stenoses exceeding 50% and above, the coincidence of both methods was 95%. The method confirms the suitability of CTA as a screening method for patients with carotid stenosis. In hemodynamically significant stenoses detected by STA screening, it appears that conventional angiography still needs to be applied [46].

The diagnostic value of CTA in a study of the Circle of Willis in patients with acute stroke was compared to MR angiography and DSA in 145 patients. CT angiograms were estimated as good or excellent in 89% of cases, and MR angiograms were estimated as such in 92% of cases. Arterial stenoses or occlusions were found in 43% of CT angiograms; they were found in 48% of MR angiograms and in 21% of DSA angiograms. The study showed that CTA is an accurate and safe method for assessing arterial stenosis and occlusion of the blood vessels in the Circle of Willis [47].

The diagnostic capabilities of CTA and MRA as noninvasive techniques were compared with DSA in 146 stroke patients. In comparison with DSA, STA and MRA showed inaccurate results in lower-grade stenosis. DSA methodology remains the gold standard in the diagnosis of patients with cerebrovascular injuries [48–50].

The role of cerebral angiography in the diagnosis of cerebrovascular diseases is sometimes questioned by the increasing importance of MR angiography. Studies in patients with atherosclerotic cerebrovascular disease have shown that MRA can almost completely displace brain angiography as a screening method for carotid bifurcation. However, the discovery of "pseudo-occlusion" still requires the use of digital subtraction angiography for accurate diagnosis. DSA is more indicative in detecting distal artery occlusions. Subarachnoid hemorrhage, detected by computed tomography, must necessarily be examined by cerebral angiography, although magnetic resonance angiography may be used as a screening test for aneurysms larger than 3 mm. The cerebral angiography is still indispensable in confirming the diagnosis of cerebrovascular malformations, arterial dissection, and fibromuscular dysplasia [51, 52].

A significant number of patients with cerebral transient ischemic accidents develop ischemic stroke in the first few months and years. A multicenter clinical trial was conducted among 3886 patients who had had transient ischemic accidents with the aim of assessing the risk of developing an early stroke. Risk factors for cerebrovascular disease (high blood pressure, age, diabetes mellitus, carotid stenoses, etc.) were studied. Instrumental methods such as magnetic resonance tomography and Doppler ultrasound were used. The results were assessed by a point system. The authors recommend new studies to be conducted, aiming at verification of the use of the methods applied [53].

Outpatient diagnosis is an important initial step in emergency treatment of stroke. A number of screening tests have been developed to identify patients at high risk of stroke. Early transportation of the patient to the hospital allows thrombolysis to be administered and improves prognosis for the final outcome of the disease [54].

Symptoms, related to the damage to the internal and external carotid arteries, were investigated, and a clinical analysis of the progressive cerebral infarction was performed in 248 patients (142 men and 106 women, average age 67.2 years). Two groups of 60 patients with progressive and 188 patients with nonprogressive cerebral infarction, respectively, were formed, the infarctions having occurred as a result of mild, moderate, and severe carotid stenoses. All patients were examined with Doppler sonography, computed or magnetic resonance tomography. Some risk factors for cerebrovascular disease (hypertonic disease, smoking, alcohol abuse, hyperlipidemia, etc.) were studied.

Since carotid arteries are the major source of blood for the brain, intima-media increased thickness is a sign of early atherosclerosis, which gradually progresses. Thrombotic and embolic processes, as well as cerebral transient ischemic accidents, are often developed with a subsequent cerebral infarction. Studies have shown that the amount of atheromatous plaques in the carotid arteries is essential for the development of severe stenoses and hemodynamic disorders in the brain. At this stage, the treatment of progressive cerebral infarction is conducted with antiaggregants, fibrinolytic agents, etc., and in some cases, endarterectomy is administered, especially in severe stenoses of the carotid arteries. Doppler ultrasound exam of extra- and intracranial vessels should be conducted within the first 24 h of the onset of the vascular accident, followed by subsequent dynamic observation.

Ischemic stroke and cerebral transient ischemic accidents are clinical diagnoses for the confirmation of which, as well as for the exclusion of cerebral hemorrhage, computed tomography and magnetic resonance tomography of the brain are performed. MRT is a more sensitive method but is often not available especially in smaller hospitals. In a clinical study in Australia, it was shown that the mean time (IQR) from hospital arrival to brain scanning should be 1.8 h (0.9–3.6 h); in this case, only 51% of the patients had their brain examined within 4.5 h of stroke. In addition, these patients should also be tested with Doppler ultrasound and electrocardiography.

Emergency diagnostics is also needed for the timely inclusion of thrombolytic therapy with RT-PA [24, 55].

5. Differences in the incidence of carotid stenoses by gender

Gender plays an important role in cardiovascular disease. Epidemiologic studies have demonstrated that men have a higher incidence and prevalence rate of stroke than women. The strokes that do occur in women tend to be more severe, however. In terms of revascularization, the available literature suggests that women have higher risk of perioperative adverse events. This thus puts into question how much women actually benefit from carotid revascularization compared with men.

The available literature suggests that women have a higher risk of perioperative adverse events during carotid revascularization. In the Asymptomatic Carotid Atherosclerosis Study (ACAS), women had a higher rate of perioperative events (3.6 vs. 1.7% for men) during CEA. Combining that with a lower rate of events for women (8.7 vs. 12.1% for men) treated with best medical therapy, this led to a much lower 5-year risk reduction for women (17%) compared with men (66%). Among patients with moderate stenosis in the North American Symptomatic Carotid Endarterectomy Trial (NASCET), the number needed to treat with CEA to prevent one ipsilateral stroke was 12 and the number needed to treat to prevent one disabling stroke was 16 for men. The corresponding numbers for women were 67 and 125, respectively, potentially suggesting a lower long-term benefit of surgery for women. The Asymptomatic Carotid Surgery Trial (ACST) produced similar findings, with men deriving a higher 5-year absolute risk reduction (8.21 vs. 4.08%) than women.

The data are somewhat unclear in the recent trials evaluating CAS and CEA. Women in the International Carotid Stenting Study (ICSS) had a higher 120-day event rate for CEA (7.6 vs. 4.2%) but a lower rate for CAS (8.0 vs. 8.7%). The opposite was found in the Carotid Revascularization Endarterectomy vs. Stenting Trial (CREST), with a lower periprocedural event rate for women undergoing CEA (3.8%) than men (4.9%) but higher in CAS (6.8 vs. 4.3%). With potentially higher perioperative event rates, these data raise the question of how much women actually benefit from intervention [50].

A database of 938 carotid arteriogram entries was established prospectively, with accompanying measurements of peak systolic velocity (PSV) and end-diastolic velocity (EDV). The percent of internal carotid artery stenosis seen on arteriograms was calculated according to criteria from the North American Symptomatic Carotid Endarterectomy Trial. Analyses were made in 536 carotid arteries in men and 402 carotid arteries in women. In addition, the single most diseased artery per patient was analyzed by gender. PSV and EDV were averaged for data subsets according to 10% intervals of internal carotid artery stenoses. Velocity for each interval was compared between men and women with the Student *t* test. Receiver operator characteristic curves were developed to define optimal duplex criteria for 60 and 70% stenosis.

For all intervals, PSV and EDV averaged 9 and 6% higher, respectively, in women than in men. Significant gender differences existed between PSV and EDV for 60 and 70% stenosis. When a single vessel per patient was analyzed, these observations persisted, but lost significance for PSV at 60% stenosis. Receiver operator characteristic curves at 90% sensitivity demonstrated that optimal PSV for 60% stenosis was 160 and 180 cm/s, and for 70% stenosis was 185 and 202 cm/s, in male and female patients, respectively.

Women have higher carotid blood flow velocity than men do. Gender differences exist and are notably different at clinically relevant thresholds for intervention. These data indicate that different criteria should be used for interpreting carotid velocity profiles in women than in men and have potentially important implications for patient care [5].

We examined 974 subjects aged 25–88 years (478 men and 496 women) in whom we considered heart rate, smoking status, and the presence of hypertension, diabetes, hypercholesterolemia, and hypertriglyceridemia. Ultrasound examination of the neck vessels included measurement of intimal medial thickness (IMT), vessel diameter, and outflow area/inflow area ratio. We established plaque location, echogenicity and echostructure, and the percentage of stenosis owing to plaque and measured systolic velocity, flow direction, and the depth of detection of these parameters. We used the apnea and hyperpnea test to assess cerebrovascular reactivity. Hypertension and hypercholesterolemia were the most frequent risk factors. Women had a higher heart rate, whereas men had significantly greater IMT. The presence of atheromatous plaque was significantly correlated with age in both sexes, with men having a higher prevalence of carotid plaques. The sexes differed significantly with regard to plaque location, echogenicity, echostructure, and intracranial circulation. Women had a slightly higher blood flow velocity in the intracranial arteries. Risk factors affected plaque formation and extent more in men than in women. These findings suggest that carotid stenosis is a gender-related trait [47].

High-resolution Doppler ultrasonography of 500 carotid bifurcations was performed in 192 women and 308 men before surgical treatment. Carotid stenoses averaged 70 ± 11% (30–95%) in women and 72 ± 12% (40–98%) in men. The prevalence of 90–99% stenosis was greater in men, 14.3 vs. 7.8%. Carotid plaques were longer in men, 2.3 ± 0.8 vs. 1.9 ± 0.6 cm. Mean diameters of the distal internal carotid artery, 4.9 ± 0.9 vs. 4.6 ± 0.8 mm, and of the common carotid artery, 7.6 ± 1.3 vs. 7.1 ± 1.4 mm, were greater in men. The distance from the ear lobe to the bifurcation was also greater in men, 5.9 ± 1.1 vs. 5.3 ± 0.9 cm. Doppler ultrasonography preoperative mapping demonstrated that the parameters measured were greater in men than in women. Detailed planning of carotid plaque treatment must take into consideration individual differences such as those associated with the patient's gender [36].

6. Conclusion

The large number of diagnostic methods and combinations of these allow early and accurate diagnosis of carotid diseases. However, it is not possible in the day-to-day practice to apply several of them at the same time. The combination of noncontrast computed tomography of the brain with Doppler ultrasound exam of the neck and head vessels in most cases provides sufficient data both for morphological changes in brain tissue and for various carotid stenoses, which are one of the well-documented risk factors for cerebrovascular disease.

Author details

Lachezar Manchev

Address all correspondence to: lachezar_manchev@yahoo.it

Faculty of Medicine, Department of Radiology, Trakia University, Stara Zagora, Bulgaria

References

[1] Шотеков П. Ултразвуково изследване на каротидните артерии. В кн. Патология на каротидната артерия (ред. П.Шотеков). София: АРСО; 2008:107-148

[2] Шотеков П. Ултразвукова диагноза на атеросклеротичните плаки. В кн. Патология на каротидната артерия (ред. П.Шотеков). София: АРСО; 2008:148-155

[3] Adams GJ, Simoni DM, Bordelon CB, et al. Bilateral symmetry of human carotid artery atherosclerosis. Stroke. 2002;**33**:2575-2580

[4] Alexandrov AV, Feldberg RA, Demchuk AM, et al. Deterioration following spontaneous improvement: Sonographic findings in patients with acutely resolving symptoms of cerebral ischemia. Stroke. 2000;**31**:915-919

[5] Carroll BA. Duplex sonography in patients with hemispheric symptoms. Journal of Ultrasound in Medicine. 1989;**8**:535-540

[6] Grant EG, Benson CB, Moneta GL, et al. Carotid artery stenosis: Gray-scale and Doppler US diagnosis—Society of Radiologists in Ultrasound Consensus Conference. Radiology. 2003;**229**:340-346

[7] Tsivgoulis G, Sharma VK, Lao AY, et al. Validation of transcranial Doppler with computed tomography angiography in acute cerebral ischemia. Stroke. 2007;**38**:1245-1249

[8] Daskalov I. Ultrasonic diagnostic. Medical instrumention. Sofia: TEMPUS BAN (Biomedical Engineering Laboratory); 1995

[9] Ringelstein EB. A practical guide to transcranial Doppler sonography. In: Noninvasive Imaging of Cerebrovascular Disease. New York: AR Liss; 1989. p. 75

[10] Baumgartner RW. Handbook on neurovascular ultrasound. Frontiers of Neurology and Neuroscience. Basel, Karger; 2006. pp. 276-283

[11] Sliwka U, Klotzsch C, Popescu O, et al. Chronic middle cerebral artery stenoses represent an embolic focus. Stroke. 1997;**28**:1324-1327

[12] Demchuk AM, Burgin WS, Cristou I, et al. Thrombolysis in brain ischemia (TIBI) transcranial Doppler flow grades predict clinical severity, early recovery and mortality in patients treated with intravenous tissue plasminogen activator. Stroke. 2001;**32**:89-93

[13] Krejza J, Owlasink M, Fryc J, et al. Transcranial color Doppler sonography in the emergency diagnosis of middle cerebral artery occlusion in patients after head injury. Mendeley. **25**(2):90-94

[14] Bartels E. Farbduplexsonographie der hirnversorgenden Gefasse. Atlas und Handbuch. Stuttgart, New York: Schatauer Verlag GmbH; 1999

[15] Reutern GM, Budingen HJ. Ultrasound Diagnosis of Cerebrovascular Disease. Doppler Sonography of the Extra- and Intracranial Arteries. Duplex Scanning. Stuttgart, NY: G. Thieme; 1993

[16] Budingen HJ, Reutern GM. Frend Doppler-Sonographie der Extracraniallen. Stuttgart: Thieme; 1982

[17] Шотеков П. Ултразвукови методи за изследване на мозъчните артерии. В кн. Патология на каротидната артерия (ред. П.Шотеков). София: АРСО; 2008:58-83

[18] Anderson GB, Ashforth R, Steinke DE, et al. CT angiography for the detection and characterization of carotid artery bifurcation disease. Stroke. 2000;**31**:2168-2174

[19] Lecrerc X, Godefroy O, Pruvo JP, et al. Computed tomographic angiography for the evaluation of carotid artery stenosis. Stroke. 1995;**26**:1577-1581

[20] Matsumoto M, Kodama N, Sakuma J, et al. 3D-CT arteriography and 3D-CT venography: The separate demonstration of arterial-phase and venous-phase on 3D-CT angiography in a single procedure. American Journal of Neuroradiology. 2005;**26**:635-641

[21] Verro P, Tonenbaum LN, Borden NM, et al. CT angiography in acute ischemic stroke: Preliminary results. Stroke. 2002;**33**:276-278

[22] Bradley WG. Magnetic Resonance Imaging. 3rd ed. St.Louis: Mosby-Year Book; 1999

[23] Kallmes DF, Omary RA, Dix JE, et al. Specificity of MR angiography as a confirmatory test of carotid artery stenosis. American Journal of Neurology. 1996;**17**:1501-1506

[24] The European Stroke Organisation (ESO) Executive Committee and the ESO Writing Committee. National Stroke Association. Guidelines for management of ischaemic stroke and transient ischaemic attack. Cerebrovascular Diseases. 2008;**25**:457-507

[25] Bakshi R, Alexandrov AV, Gomez C, et al. Neuroimaging Curriculum for Neurology Trainees: Report from the Neuroimaging Section of the AAN. American Academy of Neurology. Journal of Neuroimaging. 1999;**1**:1347-1356

[26] Fiebach J, Jansen O, Schellinger P, et al. Comparison of CT with diffusion-weighted MRI in patients with hyperacute stroke. Neuroradiology. 2001;**43**:628-632

[27] Fiebach JB, Schellinger PD, Jansen O, et al. CT and diffusion-weighted MR imaging in randomized order: Diffusion-weighted imaging results in higher accuracy and lower interrater variability in the diagnosis of hyperacute ischemic stroke. Stroke. 2002;**33**: 2206-2210

[28] Katz DA, Marks MP, Napel SA, et al. Circle of Willis: Evaluation with spiral CT angiography, MR angiography and conventional angiography. Radiology. 1995;**195**: 445-449

[29] Lubezky N, Fajer S, Barmeir E, et al. Duplex scanning and CT angiography in the diagnosis of carotid artery occlusion: A prospective study. European Journal of Vascular and Endovascular Surgery. 1998;**16**:133-136

[30] Seemann MD, Engimeer RH, Schuhmann RG, et al. Evaluation of the carotid and vertebral arteries; comparison of 3D SCTA and IA-DSA-work in progress. European Radiology. 1998;**9**(1):105-112

[31] Herzig R, Bulval S, Krupka B. Comparison of ultrasonography, CT angiography, and digital subtraction angiography in severe carotis stenosis. European Journal of Neurology. 2004;**11**:774-781

[32] Schellinger PD, Richter G, Kormann M, et al. Noninvasive angiography (magnetic resonance and computed tomography) in the diagnosis of ischemic cerebrovascular disease. Cerebrovascular Diseases. 2007;**24**(1):16-23

[33] Klingebiel R, Busch M, Zimmer C, et al. Multi-slice CT angiography in the evaluation of patients with acute cerebrovascular disease—A promising new diagnostic tool. Journal of Neurology. 2001;**249**(1):43-49

[34] Ringelstein EB, Zeumer H, Poeck K. Noninvasive diagnosis of intracranial lesions in the vertebrobasilar system: A comparison of Doppler sonographic and angiographic findings. Stroke. 1985;**16**:848-855

[35] Demchuk AM, Cristou I, Wein TH, et al. Specific transcranial Doppler flow findings related to the presence and site of arterial occlusion. Stroke. 2000;**31**:140-146

[36] Mullges W, Ringelstein EB, Leibold M. Non-invasive diagnosis of internal carotid artery dissections. Journal of Neurology, Neurosurgery, and Psychiatry. 1992;**55**:98-104

[37] Bojinova V. Clinical manifestations of cerebrovascular hypoplasias in childhood. Journal of Child Neurology. 2000;**15**(3):166-171

[38] Brandt T, Knauth M, Wildermuth S, et al. CT angiography and Doppler sonography for emergency assessment in acute basilar artery ischemia. Stroke. 1999;**30**:606-612

[39] Binaghi S, Maeder P, Uske A, et al. Three-dimensional computed tomography, angiography and magnetic resonance angiography of carotid bifurcation stenosis. European Neurology. 2001;**46**:25-34

[40] Moll R, Dinkel HP. Value of the CT angiography in the diagnosis of common carotid artery bifurcation disease: CT angiography versus digital subtraction angiography and color flow Doppler. European Journal of Radiology. 2001;**39**(3):155-163

[41] Suwanwela NC, Phanthumchinda K, Suwanrela N. Transcranial Doppler sonography and CT angiography in patients with atherothrombotic middle cerebral artery stroke. American Journal of Neuroradiology. 2002;**23**:1352-1355

[42] Wong KS, Liang EY, Lam WW, et al. Spiral computed tomography angiography in the assessment of middle cerebral artery occlusive disease. Journal of Neurology, Neurosurgery, and Psychiatry. 1995;**59**:537-539

[43] Brunster AM, Lavados PM, Hoppe A. Accuracy of transcranial Doppler compared with CT angiography in diagnosing arterial obstructions in acute ischemic strokes. Stroke. 2009;**40**:2037-2041

[44] Brossmann M, Link J, Grabener M, et al. Spiral CT angiography and selected digital subtraction angiography of internal carotid artery stenosis. American Journal of Neuroradiology. 1996;**17**:89-94

[45] Josephson SA, Bryant SO, Mak HK, et al. Evaluation of carotid stenosis using CT angiography in the initial evaluation of stroke and TIA. Neurology. 2004;**63**(3):457-460

[46] Berg M, Zhang Z, Ikonen A, et al. Multi-detector row CT angiography in the assessment of carotid artery disease in symptomatic patients: Comparison with subtraction angiography. American Journal of Neuroradiology. 2005;**26**:1022-1034

[47] Shrier DA, Tanaka H, Numaguchi Y, et al. CT-angiography in the evaluation of acute stroke. American Journal of Neuroradiology. 1997;**18**:1011-1020

[48] Alvarez-Linera J, Benito-Leon J, Escribano J, et al. Prospective evaluation of carotid artery stenosis: Elliptic centric contrast-enhanced MR angiography and spiral CT angiography compared with digital subtraction angiography. American Journal of Neuroradiology. 2003;**24**:1012-1019

[49] Biffl WL, Ray CE, Moore EE, et al. Noninvasive diagnosis of blunt cerebrovascular injuries. A preliminary report. Journal of Trauma-Injury Infectional Critical Care. 2002; **53**:850-856

[50] Hirai T, Korogi Y, Ono K, et al. Prospective evaluation of suspected stenooclusive disease of the intracranial artery: Combined MR angiography and CT angiography compared with digital subtraction angiography. American Journal of Neuroradiology. 2002;**23**:93-101

[51] Cumming MJ, Morrow IM. Carotid artery stenosis: A prospective comparison of CT angiography and conventional angiography. American Journal of Roentgenology. 1994; **163**:517-523

[52] Villablanca JP, Martin N, Jahan R, et al. Volume-rendering helical computed tomography angiography in the detection and characterization of intracranial aneurysms. Journal of Neurosurgery. 2000;**93**:254-264

[53] Merwick A, Albers GW, Amarenko P, et al. Addition of brain and carotid imaging to the ABCD score to identify patients at early risk of stroke after transient ischaemic attack: A multicentre observational study. Lancet Neurology. 2010;**9**:1060-1069

[54] Rae V, Ford G, Price C. Prehospital assessment of stroke: Time is brain. Journal of Paramedic Practice. 2011;**3**(9):483-488

[55] National Stroke Audit Acute Services. Clinical Audit Report, Melbourne, Australia; 2011. pp. 21-27

Chapter 4

Flow Velocity in Common Carotid Artery

A. Rahman Rasyada and Azran Azhim

Additional information is available at the end of the chapter

http://dx.doi.org/10.5772/intechopen.80712

Abstract

A significant blood flow disruption as seen in cardiovascular diseases and disorders is related to hemodynamic dysfunction. Gender influences the arterial hemodynamic functions. Understanding of gender-related differences in blood flow and pressure is crucial in the prevalence and burden of cardiovascular disease. This chapter presents about characteristic profile of carotid flow velocities to extend the fundamental understanding of arterial hemodynamic functions in gender differences. Comparison of both synchronized carotid blood flow velocity and blood pressures at normodynamics state are introduced to contribute to targeted therapeutic goal based on gender. Gender-related differences in body size has influenced on arterial hemodynamics in carotid artery. Body height has influenced on systolic blood pressure, pulse pressure, wave reflection, pulse wave velocity in carotid artery. Carotid blood flow velocities are largely accounted for not only body height but also body weight. The predictors for modulating blood flow velocities were not only limited to age, but also influenced by several body compositions that largely accounted for the gender-related differences including visceral fat, muscle mass and total body fat. These data may useful to effective prevention and management of cardiovascular disease by considering the gender-difference.

Keywords: flow velocity, common carotid artery, health, gender, body composition

1. Introduction

Hemodynamic is dealing with blood flow and forces concerned therein to circulate blood through the cardiovascular system. A significant blood flow disruption as seen in cardiovascular diseases and disorders is related to hemodynamic dysfunction. Doppler ultrasound has potential to serve as a non-invasive method for detecting and quantifying blood flow functions in cardiovascular diseases. However, the use of blood flow in clinical application is limited and development of blood flow is prevailing rather than blood flow [1].

Gender influences the arterial hemodynamic functions. Cardiovascular disease is a leading cause of death for both women and men, but there are crucial gender-related differences in the prevalence and burden of cardiovascular disease. An approach to understand this disparity is to evaluate the underlying changes in hemodynamic functions and discover the relationship between the gender differences and cardiovascular disease risk. Gender-related differences in systolic blood pressure (SBP) are reported in previous studies [2, 3]. It is widely reported that gender differences in blood pressures (i.e. SBP and pulse pressure) and arterial wave reflections are associated to smaller body height of women [4–6].

Azhim et al. have developed a Doppler measurement system to evaluate flow velocity functions in common carotid artery with synchronized monitoring of blood pressure (BP) and electrocardiogram (ECG) [6, 7]. Firstly, this chapter presents about characteristic profile of carotid flow velocities in an attempt to extend the fundamental understanding of arterial hemodynamic functions in gender differences. Secondly, comparison of carotid flow velocity and other parameters at resting posture in gender are introduced. The extent to which body size including body height and weight have influenced on blood velocities in carotid artery is described in Section 3. Furthermore, the blood flow velocity also useful for comparing the effect of fat compositions in gender differences as presented in Section 4.

2. Normohemodynamics in gender

In hemodynamics studies, abnormality of blood flow can be detected from Doppler waveforms, vascular structure and function may be identified through various quantitative measurements made [1, 8]. This section does not focus on hemodynamic disorders, aging, and response to exercise or during exercise. But, the findings do fill important literature gap in correlation between gender-related differences with hemodynamic variables. The normohemodynamics of carotid artery and other parameters are determined in healthy sedentary subjects to rule out the effects that exercise may have on the dependent variables. From a total of 85 sedentary subjects, 49 of them are men.

The Doppler frequency shift represents temporal changes in peak velocities of blood cells movement during particular cardiac cycle. Several analytic techniques have been proposed for analyzing the velocity waveform. Most of these techniques involve analysis of maximum velocity at particular points on Doppler waveforms described as peak velocity envelope. By using the developed measurement system by Azhim et al., carotid blood flow velocity was measured simultaneously with commercialized ECG by three-leads and brachial BP [6, 7]. Measurements of ECG and BP were used as reference data. To extract peak velocity values from its velocity spectra, a threshold method and computation using ensemble averaging technique was implemented in this study. As shown in **Figure 1**, 30 consecutive cardiac cycles were selected from 2 minutes spectral to characterize the feature points of peak velocity envelope and calculate its indices. In this study, flow velocities in carotid artery were characterized into five feature points [9, 10]. The first peak systolic velocity wave was peak velocity S1. It represents the maximum velocity during systole. Consequently it is usually used as an ejection parameter in cardiac systole [11]. An augmented velocity in late systole wave was the

http://dx.doi.org/10.5772/intechopen.80712

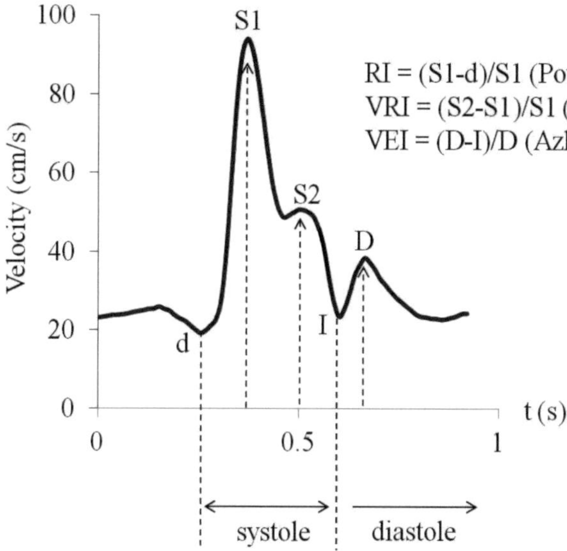

Figure 1. Doppler indices derived from peak systolic velocity (S1), second systolic (S2), insicura between systole and diastole (I), peak diastolic (D) and end-diastolic (d) velocities.

second systolic velocity S2. Augmentation of S2 was related to both reflection of pulse wave velocity at branching site and reflection of pressure wave [1, 9]. The peak diastolic velocity, D velocity was the maximum velocity which rises due vascular elastic recoil during cardiac diastole, insicura between systole and diastole (I) [9] and the end-diastolic velocity, d represents the minimum velocity during diastole [9, 11].

Usually blood velocity indices or ratios were derived from various combinations of the peak systolic velocity, end-diastolic velocity, and temporal mean values of the maximum Doppler frequency shift envelope [11, 12]. Of various indices, resistance index (RI) has been used extensively to measure the pulsatility that reflects the resistance to blood flow [12]. RI has defined range limit which is between value of 0–1.0. It was suggested to be used for analyzing waveforms with continuous forward flow throughout the diastole such as in carotid artery [8]. Unlike S1/d ratio as developed by Stuart and Drumm [13], RI shows Gaussian distribution and therefore can be analyzed through parametric statistical analyses. The RI data also reported to have better discriminatory performance compared to pulsatility index (PI) data [11]. Velocity reflection index (VRI) and velocity elastic index (VEI) were first proposed by [9] to evaluate aging and exercise effects. The VRI was a relation with S1 and S2 which calculated from (S2 − S1)/S1. The validation of VRI was analyzed using linear regression analysis. It increased with pressure reflection wave of augmentation index (r^2 = 0.836). The latter index was calculated from (D − I)/D. It corresponds to vascular elasticity properties during cardiac diastole [9] as shown in **Figure 1**. Because of the velocity features are obtained from same cardiac cycle, the indices are independent of insonation angle [11].

Rough reference of gender-related differences in hemodynamic characteristics is summarized in **Table 1**. As previously we have reported that carotid flow velocities have influenced by multiple effects including regular exercise, aging and visceral fat accumulation [7, 14–16], the

Variable	Women (n = 36)	Men (n = 49)	*p*-value
Age (years)	35.2 ± 1.9	38.4 ± 2.2	NS
Height (cm)	157.9 ± 0.9	168.8 ± 0.9	<0.01
Blood pressure data			
SBP (mmHg)	118.5 ± 2.4	129.2 ± 2.1	<0.01
DBP (mmHg)	73.7 ± 1.8	80.5 ± 1.8	<0.05
MBP (mmHg)	89.0 ± 2.0	96.7 ± 1.9	<0.01
HR (bpm)	73.8 ± 2.1	73.6 ± 1.6	NS
Flow velocity data			
d (cm/s)	23.7 ± 0.8	18.9 ± 0.7	<0.01
S1 (cm/s)	96.9 ± 3.2	91.2 ± 3.1	NS
S2 (cm/s)	64.3 ± 2.0	50.0 ± 1.8	<0.01
I (cm/s)	35.6 ± 1.3	27.5 ± 0.9	<0.01
D (cm/s)	45.6 ± 1.2	39.1 ± 1.0	<0.01
RI	0.750 ± 0.010	0.785 ± 0.009	<0.05
VRI	−0.318 ± 0.026	−0.423 ± 0.028	<0.05
VEI	0.223 ± 0.016	0.298 ± 0.017	<0.01

Data are presented as mean ± standard error of mean. The *p*-value indicates significance difference versus women. NS indicates not significant. d: end-diastolic velocity; S1: peak systolic velocity; S2: second systolic velocity; I: insicura between systole and diastole; D: peak diastolic velocity; RI: resistive index; VRI: velocity reflection index; VEI: vascular elasticity index.

Table 1. Differences in hemodynamic characteristics in women and men.

presented data of hemodynamics differences in gender are also considering the influenced effects of that. The age differences is taken into account by matching the age variable with keeping not significant mean and low standard error. The range subjects' age for men and women are 20–58 years (38.4 ± 2.2) and 20–64 years (35.2 ± 1.9) respectively. Generally men are taller than women.

Study of blood pressure to explain gender-related differences in arterial hemodynamic functions is prevailing than blood flow velocity. It has been reported that hemodynamic dysfunction increases with SBP [17]. Women have a lower SBP when measured in both brachial and ankle-arm and pressure index than age-matched men [2]. Gender-related differences in body height has influenced to arterial hemodynamics such as SBP, pulse pressure, wave reflection and pulse wave velocity in carotid artery [4, 5]. We found that the gender differences in arterial hemodynamics in carotid flow velocities are largely accounted for body height and weight [6, 7].

With increases of blood pressure in men, all velocity waveforms were homeostatically lower. Men and women have different envelope velocity waveforms in carotid artery shown in **Figure 2.** In this study, we found that women have a lower brachial SBP than men, but higher

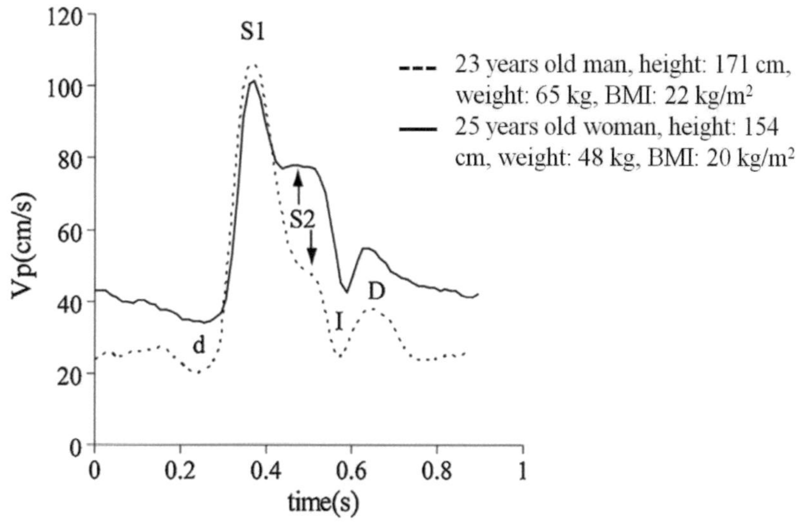

Figure 2. Comparison of typical envelope velocity waveforms in carotid artery for age-matched man (dashed line) and woman (solid line). d: end-diastolic velocity; S1: peak systolic velocity; S2: second systolic velocity; I: insicura between systole and diastole; D: peak diastolic velocity. Adapted from Azhim et al. [7].

d, S2, I and D velocities. Therefore, women have lower RI and VEI, and had higher VRI than men. Consistent with previous studies, pressure wave reflection and propagation are known to be correlated with body height [2, 3, 18], Azhim et al. also suggests that the reflected wave in flow components was higher in women and is significantly correlated with body height [7]. Men have been reported to have more elastic arterial trees than women [2, 7].

3. Arterial hemodynamic changes: role of body size

Effective regulation of blood flow and blood pressure in order to maintain homeostasis is a primary aspect of cardiovascular health. In general young women have lower resting blood pressure [19–21] and in response to physiological changing [22]. The systolic and diastolic BP increased in response to the graded, incremental tilt and the difference observed between men and women is reflective of differences in body size (i.e. in particular height) as shown in **Figure 3** [22]. Epidemiological studies based on brachial artery pressure indicate that blood pressures were lower in young women than in age-matched men [2, 6]. Generally, SBP and pulse pressure increased as a pulse travels from aorta towards the peripheral, the increase being all the more pronounced as the distance of pulse propagation [2].

Changes in velocity envelope waveforms at peak systolic velocity, augmented velocity in late systole wave (i.e. S2) and end-diastolic velocity are focused on their relationship with aging and carotid diseases [23]. Addition to S1, d velocities and its index (i.e., RI) decreasing with age, S2, D velocities and its indices (i.e., VRI and VEI) decrease continuously with age that may increase the complication in cardiovascular disease risk [7]. Only few studies have considered the latter velocities and indices in association with gender or disease [22, 24]. To the best of our knowledge, no other studies have characterized the correlations of these velocities with

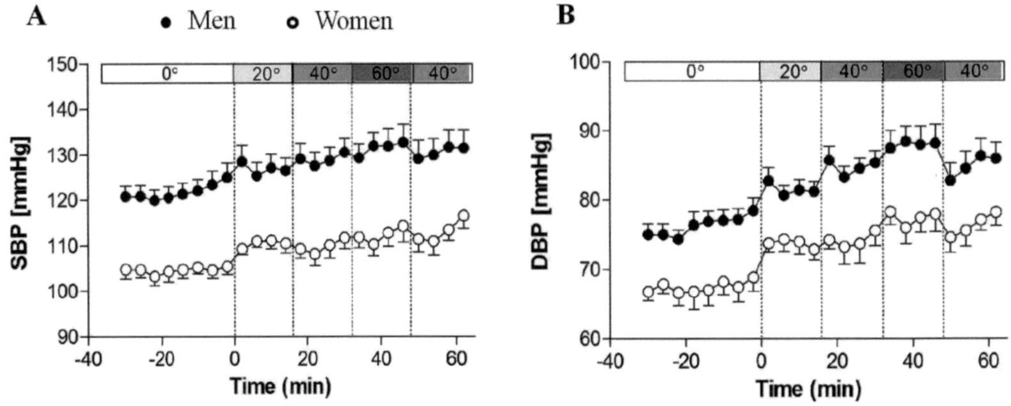

Figure 3. Blood pressure variability in response to graded, incremental tilt in healthy young men (n = 13) and women (n = 10). (A) Systolic blood pressure and (B) diastolic blood pressure. Tilt angle is indicated in the bar above each panel (i.e., 0° (resting posture), 20°, 40°, 60°, and back to 40°). Adapted from Sarafian and Miles-Chan [22].

gender, age, visceral fat accumulation and exercise [7, 16]. In this study, we found significant differences in the carotid velocity waveforms of age-matched men and women to contribute to clinical evaluations and healthcare monitoring [6].

Women had larger reflected waves than men, in part due to shorter body height and closer physical proximity between heart and reflecting sites. However, body height was not sufficient to fully explain higher reflected wave flow and pressure in women. In the study we indicated that the reflected wave had higher in women and was significantly correlated to body height and weight as described in **Figures 4** and **5** [6]. In addition to knowledge that pressure wave reflection and propagation are known to correlate with body height [2, 3], we also found that increased reflected flow wave was partially influenced by decreased body

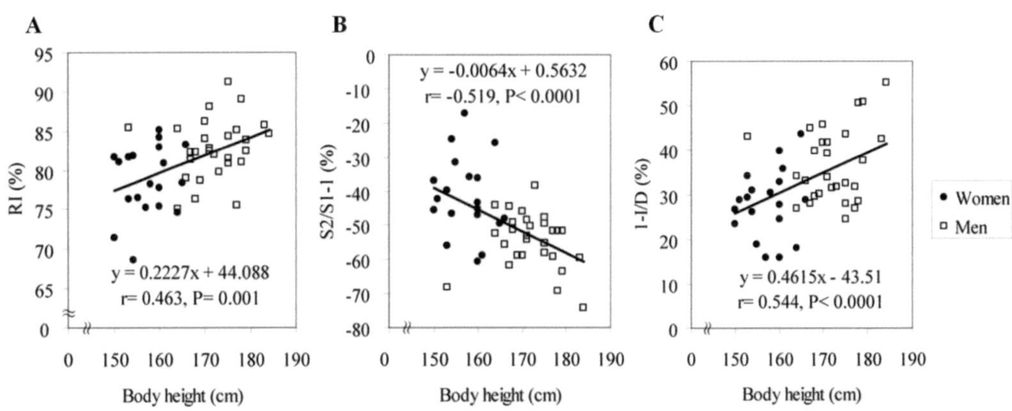

Figure 4. The velocity indices correlated with height. (A) RI: resistive index (1 – d/S1); (B) VRI: velocity reflection index (S2/S1 – 1); (C) VEI: vascular elasticity index (1 – I/D). Men (n = 30) are represented by open circles and women (n = 20) represented by closed circles. Adapted from Azhim et al. [6].

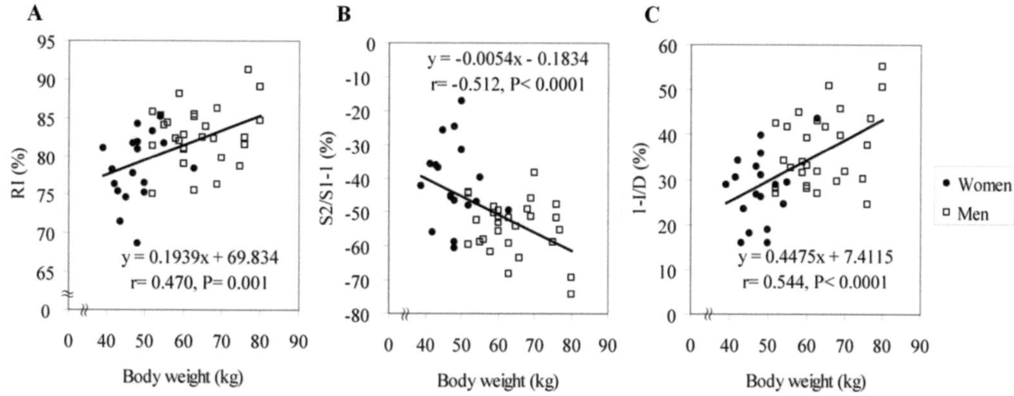

Figure 5. The velocity indices correlated with weight. (A) RI: resistive index (1 − d/S1); (B) VRI: velocity reflection index (S2/S1 − 1); (C) VEI: vascular elasticity index (1 − I/D). Men (n = 30) are represented by open circles and women (n = 20) represented by closed circles. Adapted from Azhim et al. [6].

weight and increased heart rate level [6]. It had been reported that women had lower carotid artery distensibility compared with men [25]. From the proposed velocity indices (i.e. VEI), we agreed that women had lower arterial elasticity [6, 7]. The difference in the velocities and its indices were related to smaller body size in women that largely accounted for the gender differences. The difference in velocity indices may also contributed by concentrations of estrogen in women hormone status of women [26].

4. Arterial hemodynamic changes: role of body compositions

Although the risk for cardiovascular disease increases with age, occurrence and burden of cardiovascular disease may possibly higher in men as described by differences in blood flow velocities and blood pressures [2, 7]. Furthermore body fat composition in the specific body region could explain underlying relationship between the gender-related differences and cardiovascular disease risk such as hypertension [15, 27]. Men tend to accumulate upper body fat which mainly around the abdominal area in the form visceral fat (VF), whereas women tend to have fat deposited in the gluteofemoral region [28, 29]. In the Framingham Heart Study indicated that small differences in VF among three different body mass index classifications; normal-weight, overweight or obese groups can significantly change health risk profile including hypertension [30]. It also widely known that VF increase with aging and associated with clinical features of metabolic variables including elevated triglyceride, glucose and reduced high density lipoprotein [31, 32]. The presented data in **Table 2** is to demonstrate a rough reference of gender-related differences in body compositions in sedentary healthy subjects. Men showed a greater body mass index, weight and muscle mass. An alternative to general indication of abdominal VF is waist circumference measurement. The prevalence of having higher VF and waist circumference in men was dominant. But, women showed higher total body fat.

Variable	Women (n = 36)	Men (n = 49)	*p*-Value
VF (level)	3.1 ± 0.3	8.0 ± 0.7	<0.01
Weight (kg)	52.0 ± 1.1	65.2 ± 1.5	<0.01
BMI (kg/m²)	20.8 ± 0.4	22.8 ± 3.2	<0.01
WC (cm)	72.5 ± 1.2	81.0 ± 1.3	<0.01
Total body fat (kg)	28.2 ± 0.7	19.2 ± 0.8	<0.01
Muscle mass (kg)	34.0 ± 1.1	49.7 ± 0.8	<0.01
TCho (mmol/L)	191.4 ± 6.8	194.3 ± 5.6	NS
LDL (mmol/L)	97.2 ± 7.6	109.8 ± 5.3	<0.01

Data are presented as mean ± standard error of mean. The *p*-value indicates significance difference versus women. NS indicates not significant. VF: visceral fat; BMI: body mass index; WC: waist circumference; TCho: total cholesterol; LDL: low-density lipoprotein cholesterol.

Table 2. Differences in body compositions in women and men.

Extensive research in obesity when elucidating hypertension showed that site-specific fat accumulation is more important rather than total body fat [27]. Chandra et al. demonstrated that hypertension is mainly influenced by VF accumulation compared to lower body fat and subcutaneous fat [27]. The VF is also associated to coronary heart disease and systemic arteriosclerosis [33, 34]. Consequently, VF accumulation contributed to greater aortic stiffness in older adult as measured by pulse wave velocity [35]. Comparison data of gender difference is essential to provide rough indication risk of developing health problems related to fat composition.

It is widely known from literature that rising blood pressure is associated with increased cardiovascular disease risk. Women has lower blood pressures, homeostatically higher velocity waveforms with the heart rate did not comparable different than men. The VF and age were two important determinants for increase in blood pressures in our study as shown in **Table 3**.

Variable	Predictor	β	*p*	r^2
SBP (mmHg)	Constant	107.35	<0.001	0.304
	VF (level)	1.30	0.002	
	Age (years)	0.26	0.045	
DBP (mmHg)	Constant	60.64	<0.001	0.354
	Age (years)	0.34	0.002	
	VF (level)	0.78	0.017	
MBP (mmHg)	Constant	76.21	<0.001	0.359
	Age (years)	0.31	0.005	
	VF (level)	0.95	0.005	

Beta (β) value indicates regression coefficient. The *p*-value less than 0.05 indicates predictor variable has significant association with hemodynamic variable. SBP: systolic blood pressure; DBP: diastolic blood pressure; MBP: mean blood pressure.

Table 3. Stepwise linear regression analysis of blood pressure measurements.

Similar to this study, association between VF and blood pressures is found consistently in some studies [16, 27]. Using multiple regression analysis, VF becomes superior predictor to hypertension compared to lower body fat and subcutaneous fat in other study [27]. Aging is associated with a significant increase in the prevalence of hypertension and especially of systolic hypertension in elderly [36]. Elevation of blood pressure with aging is mostly associated with structural and functional changes in the arteries like large artery stiffness [9, 37]. However, the predictors for modulating blood flow velocities were not only limited on age, but also influenced by several body compositions that largely accounted for the gender differences as presented in **Table 4**.

To evaluate the predisposing factors for flow velocity in common carotid artery, stepwise regression analysis was performed with the following parameters: age, muscle mass, VF and

Variable	Predictor	β	*p*	r^2
d (cm/s)	Constant	30.45	<0.001	0.168
	Muscle mass (kg)	−0.22	<0.001	
S1 (cm/s)	Constant	125.93	<0.001	0.355
	Age (years)	−0.87	<0.001	
S2 (cm/s)	Constant	95.36	<0.001	0.308
	Muscle mass (kg)	−0.79	<0.001	
I (cm/s)	Constant	46.55	<0.001	0.193
	Muscle mass (kg)	−0.36	<0.001	
D (cm/s)	Constant	46.98	<0.001	0.251
	VF (level)	−0.86	<0.001	
RI	Constant	0.76	<0.001	0.341
	Age (years)	−0.002	<0.001	
	Muscle mass (kg)	0.002	<0.001	
VRI	Constant	−0.58	<0.001	0.667
	Age (years)	0.01	<0.001	
	Muscle mass (kg)	−0.01	<0.001	
	Total body fat (kg)	0.004	0.045	
VEI	Constant	0.24	<0.001	0.344
	Age (years)	−0.004	<0.001	
	Muscle mass (kg)	0.004	<0.001	

Beta (β) value indicates regression coefficient. The *p*-value less than 0.05 indicates predictor variable has significant association with hemodynamic variable. d: end-diastolic velocity; S1: peak systolic velocity; S2: second systolic velocity; I: insicura between systole and diastole; D: peak diastolic velocity; RI: resistive index; VRI: velocity reflection index; VEI: vascular elasticity index.

Table 4. Stepwise linear regression analysis of blood flow velocity measurements.

total body fat. This study found that VF is an important predictor that inversely related to carotid peak diastolic velocity waveform. Using the proposed index by Azhim et al., peak diastolic velocity, D is an important feature waveform to determine arterial elasticity [7]. Consequently poor arterial elasticity is attributed by accumulation of VF [16, 32] and lower arterial elasticity through its index, VEI is observed in women compared to men. Vaidya et al. also reported the same results where postmenopausal women had lower carotid elasticity compared to matched-age men based on its carotid distensibility [38]. This study can only speculate that the difference in this index could also be influenced by the sex hormone stimulation [38].

Women had greater vascular reflection wave using the proposed index (i.e. VRI) and second systolic velocity compared with men (see **Table 1**). The augmentation of second systolic flow velocity in carotid artery was related to wave reflection arriving from the lower body or thoracic aorta [39]. The wave reflection in women was related to shorter body height that reflects shorter distance to reflecting site [2, 3]. However, body height was not fully explaining the higher VRI. Significant correlations were observed between body composition variables and VRI, with age, muscle mass and total body fat also contributing to stepwise model for VRI.

Muscle mass found to be correlated with all blood flow velocities and blood pressures, but not with S1 velocity, likely due to a greater range of muscle mass among men. Interestingly, muscle mass was a stronger predictor for the most correlated blood flow velocities and indices, except for D velocity and all blood pressures. In agreement with the findings, study of healthy adults was shown an inversely correlation between thigh muscle mass and aortic pressure from wave reflections when characterized by augmentation pressure and its index [40]. By physiology and anatomy studies, left ventricular hypertrophy was observed in women via ventricular remodeling [41, 42] and had higher systolic left ventricular chamber function compared to men [43]. These factors might contribute consistent increase in the first velocity wave during systole in women. Furthermore RI was significantly lower due to increase of S1 velocity in women (RI = 1 − d/S1).

5. Conclusion

In conclusion, monitoring of blood flow velocity and blood pressure synchronized measurements may be potential to support the assessment of some main hemodynamic functions in gender difference. A fundamental understanding of gender-related differences in arterial hemodynamics is required for effective prevention and detection of cardiovascular disease at the early stage. Women have lower brachial blood pressure components than men, but higher d, S2, I and D velocities. Therefore, women have lower resistive and vascular elastic indices and had higher velocity reflection than men. Gender difference in arterial hemodynamics in carotid velocity waveforms is largely accounted for body size in particular height and weight. Furthermore unlike blood pressures, the predictors for modulating blood flow velocity not limited on age and VF factors, but also influenced by muscle mass and total body fat. Improvable screening of health problem can be achieved by monitoring the blood flow velocity together with blood pressure measurements and considering its gender-difference to fully assessing hemodynamics function in circulatory system.

Acknowledgements

This study was partly supported by Mediprotech Co. LTD., Korea under International Sponsored Research Grant (C18-058-0231) and Ministry of Higher Education Malaysia under MyBrain15 Postgraduate Scholarship Programme.

Conflict of interest

The authors do not have any conflict of interest.

Author details

A. Rahman Rasyada[1] and Azran Azhim[2*]

*Address all correspondence to: azr2020@gmail.com

1 Department of Biotechnology, Kulliyyah of Sciences, International Islamic University Malaysia, Kuantan, Malaysia

2 Department of Biomedical Sciences, Kulliyyah of Allied Health Sciences, International Islamic University Malaysia, Kuantan, Malaysia

References

[1] Nichols WW, O'Rourke MF. McDonald's Blood Flow in Arteries: Theoretic, Experimental and Clinical Principles. 5th ed. London: Hodder Arnold; 2005

[2] London GM, Guerin AP, Pannier B, Marchais SJ, Stimpel M. Influence of sex on arterial haemodynamics and blood pressure: Role of body height. Hypertension. 1995;**26**: 514-519. DOI: 10.1161/01.HYP.26.3.514

[3] Mitchell GF, Parise H, Benjamin EJ, Larson MG, Keyes MJ, Vita JA, et al. Changes in arterial stiffness and wave reflection with advancing age in healthy men and women: The Framingham Heart Study. Hypertension. 2004;**43**:1239-1245. DOI: 10.1161/01.HYP.0000128420.01881.aa

[4] London GM, Guerin AP, Pannier B, Marchais SJ, Metivier F. Body height as a determinant of carotid pulse contour in humans. Hypertension. 1992;**10**:93-95. DOI: 10.1097/00004872-199208001-00024

[5] Marchais SJ, Guerin AP, Pannier B, Levy BI, Safar ME, London GM. Wave reflections and cardiac hypertrophy in chronic uremia: Influence of body size. Hypertension. 1993;**22**:876-883. DOI: 10.1161/01.HYP.22.6.876

[6] Azhim A, Akioka K, Akutagawa M, Hirao Y, Yoshizaki K, Obara S, et al. Effect of gender on blood flow velocities and blood pressure role of body weight and height. In: Conference Proceedings for IEEE Engineering in Medicine and Biology Society. 2007. pp. 967-970. DOI: 10.1109/IEMBS.2007.4352453

[7] Azhim A, Ueno A, Tanaka M, Masatake A, Kinouchi Y. Evaluation of blood flow velocity envelope in common carotid artery for reference data. Biomedical Signal Processing and Control. 2011;**6**:209-215. DOI: 10.1016/j.bspc.2010.11.002

[8] Oates C. Cardiovascular Haemodynamics and Doppler Waveforms Explained. 1st ed. London: Greenwich Medical Media Ltd.; 2001

[9] Azhim A, Katai M, Akutagawa M, Hirao Y, Yoshizaki K, Obara S, et al. Exercise improved age-associated changes in the carotid blood velocity waveforms. Journal of Biomedical and Pharmaceutical Engineering. 2007;**1**(1):17-26

[10] Azhim A, Akutagawa M, Hirao Y. Measurement of blood flow velocity waveforms in the carotid, brachial and femoral arteries during head-up tilt. Journal of Biomedical and Pharmaceutical Engineering. 2008;**2**:1-6. DOI: 10.1109/ICBPE.2006.348631

[11] Maulik D. Spectral Doppler sonography: Waveform analysis and hemodynamic Interpretation. In: Maulik D, editor. Doppler Ultrasound in Obstetrics and Gynecology. Berlin: Springer; 2005

[12] Pourcelot L. Diagnostic ultrasound for cerebral vascular diseases. In: Donald I, Levi S, editors. Present and Future of Diagnostic Ultrasound. Rotterdam: Kooyker; 1976

[13] Stuart B, Drumm J, Fitz Gerald DE, Diugnan NM. Fetal blood velocity waveforms in normal pregnancy. British Journal of Obstetrics and Gynaecology. 1980;**87**:780-785. DOI: 10.1111/j.1471-0528.1980.tb04613.x/full

[14] Azhim A, Kinouchi Y. Portable Blood Flow Velocimetry for Health Care Monitoring. Deutschland: Lap Lambert Academic Publishing; 2014

[15] Rasyada AR, Zulaika H, Akutagawa M, Emoto T, Kinouchi Y, Azhim A. The impact of visceral fat and blood flow velocity in hypertensive subjects. Health Science Journal. 2016;**10**(2):1-6

[16] Rasyada AR, Sha'ban M, Azhim A. Influence of visceral fat and hypertension on changes of blood flow velocity in non-obese individual. Cardiovascular Journal of Africa. 2018;**29**(3):141-144. DOI: 10.5830/CVJA-2018-001

[17] Kannel WB, Stokes J. Hypertension as a cardiovascular risk factor. In: Robertson JIS editor. Handbook of Hypertension. Clinical Aspects of Hypertension. New York: Elsevier Science Publishing Co; 1985

[18] Latham RD, Westerhof N, Sipkema P, Rubal BJ, Reuderink P, Murgo JP. Regional wave travel and reflections along the human aorta: A study with six simultaneous micromanometric pressures. Circulation. 1985;**72**:1257-1269. DOI: 10.1161/01

[19] Robertson D. The epidemic of orthostatic tachycardia and orthostatic intolerance. American Journal of the Medical Sciences. 1999;**317**:75-77. DOI: 10.1016/S0002-9629(15)40480-X

[20] Waters WW, Ziegler MG, Meck JV. Postspaceflight orthostatic hypotension occurs mostly in women and is predicted by low vascular resistance. Journal of Applied Physiology. 2002;**92**:586-594. DOI: 10.1152/japplphysiol.00544.2001

[21] Fu Q, Arbab-Zadeh A, Perhonen MA, Zhang R, Zuckerman JH, Levine BD. Hemodynamics of orthostatic intolerance: Implications for gender differences. American Journal of Physiology Heart and Circulatory Physiology. 2004;**286**:449-457. DOI: 10.1152/ajpheart.00735.2002

[22] Sarafian D, Miles-Chan JL. The influence of gender and anthropometry on haemodynamic status at rest and in response to graded incremental head-up tilt in young, healthy adults. Frontiers in Physiology. 2017;**7**(656):1-10. DOI: 10.3389/fphys.2016.00656

[23] Nagatomo I, Nomaguchi M, Matsumoto K. Blood flow velocity waveform in the common carotid artery and its analysis in elderly subjects. Clinical Autonomic Research. 1992;**2**(3):197-200. PMID: 1498566

[24] Rutherford RB, Hiatt WR, Kreuter EW. The use of velocity wave form analysis in the diagnosis of carotid artery occlusive. Surgery. 1977;**82**(5):695-702. PMID: 918858

[25] Ylitalo A, Airaksinen KEJ, Hautanen A, Kupari M, Carson M, Virolainen J, et al. Baroreflex sensitivity and variants of the renin angiotensin system genes. Journal of American College of Cardiology. 2000;**35**:194-200. DOI: 10.1016/S0735-1097(99)00506-9

[26] Krejza J, Mariak Z, Huba M, Wolczynski S, Lewko J. Effect of endogenous estrogen on blood flow through carotid arteries. Stroke. 2001;**32**:30-36. DOI: 10.1161/01.STR.32.1.30

[27] Chandra A, Neeland IJ, Berry JD, Ayers CR, Rohatgi A, Das SR, et al. The relationship of body mass and fat distribution with incident hypertension; observations from the Dallas heart study. Journal of the American College of Cardiology. 2014;**64**(10):997-1002. DOI: 10.1016/j.jacc.2014.05.057

[28] Despres JP, Moorjani S, Lupien PJ, Tremblay A, Nadeau A, Bouchard C. Regional distribution of body fat, plasma lipoproteins, and cardiovascular disease. Arteriosclerosis. 1990;**10**:497-511. PMID: 2196040

[29] Lemieux S, Prud'homme D, Bouchard C, Tremblay A, Despres JP. Sex differences in the relation of visceral adipose tissue accumulation to total body fatness. American Society for Clinical Nutrition. 1993;**58**:463-467. DOI: 10.1093/ajcn/58.4.463

[30] Fox CS, Massaro JM, Hoffmann U, Pou KM, Maurovich-Horvat P, Liu CY, et al. Abdominal visceral and subcutaneous adipose tissue compartments: Association with metabolic risk factors in the Framingham Heart Study. Circulation. 2007;**116**(1):39-48. DOI: 10.1161/CIRCULATIONAHA.106.675355

[31] Francque S, Verrijken A, Mertens I, Hubens G, Marck EV, Pelckmans P, et al. Visceral adiposity and insulin resistance are independent predictors of the presence of non-cirrhotic NAFLD-related portal hypertension. International Journal of Obesity. 2011;**35**:270-278. DOI: 10.1038/ijo.2010.134

[32] Yamauchi T, Kuno T, Takada H, Nagura Y, Kanmatsuse K, Takahashi S. The impact of visceral fat on multiple risk factors and carotid atherosclerosis in chronic haemodialysis patients. Nephrology Dialysis Transplantation. 2003;**18**(9):1842-1847. DOI: 10.1093/ndt/gfg261

[33] Matsuzawa Y, Nakamura T, Shimomura I, Kotani K. Visceral fat accumulation and cardiovascular disease. Obesity. 1995;**3**(5):645-647. DOI: 10.1002/j.1550-8528.1995.tb00481.x

[34] Matsuzawa Y, Funahashi T, Nakamura T. The concept of metabolic syndrome: Contribution of visceral fat accumulation and its molecular mechanism. Journal of Atherosclerosis and Thrombosis. 2011;**18**(8):629-639. DOI: 10.5551/jat.7922

[35] Sutton-Tyrrell K, Newman A, Simonsick EM, Havlik R, Pahor M, Lakatta E, et al. Aortic stiffness is associated with visceral adiposity in older adults enrolled in the study of health, aging and body composition. Hypertension. 2001;**38**:429-433. DOI: 10.1161/01.HYP.38.3.429

[36] Anderson GH. Effect of age on hypertension: Analysis of over 4,800 referred hypertensive patients. Saudi Journal of Kidney Diseases and Transplantation. 1999;**10**(3):286-297. PMID: 18212439

[37] Pinto E. Blood pressure and ageing. Postgraduate Medical Journal. 2007;**83**:109-114. DOI: 10.1136/pgmj.2006.048371

[38] Vaidya D, Golden SH, Haq N, Heckbert SR, Liu K, Ouyang P. The association of sex hormones with carotid artery distensibility in men and postmenopausal women: Multi-ethnic study of atherosclerosis. Hypertension. 2015;**65**(5):1020-1025. DOI: 10.1161/HYPERTENSIONAHA.114.04826

[39] Heffernan KS, Lefferts WK, Augustine JA. Hemodynamic correlates of late systolic flow velocity augmentation in the carotid artery. International Journal of Hypertension. 2013;**2013**:1-7. DOI: 10.1155/2013/920605

[40] Loenneke JP, Christopher A, Fahs CA, Heffernan KS, Rossow LM, Thiebaud RS, et al. Relationship between thigh muscle mass and augmented pressure from wave reflections in healthy adults. European Journal of Applied Physiology. 2013;**113**:395-401. DOI: 10.1007/s00421-012-2449-y

[41] Carroll JD, Carroll EP, Feldman T, Ward DM, Lang RM, McGaughey D, et al. Sex-associated differences in left ventricular function in aortic stenosis of the elderly. Circulation. 1992;**86**:1099-1107. DOI: 10.1161/01.CIR.86.4.1099

[42] Krumholz HM, Larson M, Levy D. Sex differences in cardiac adaptation to isolated systolic hypertension. American Journal of Cardiology. 1993;**72**(3):310-313. DOI: 10.1016/0002-9149(93)90678-6

[43] Hayward CS, Kalnins WV, Kelly RP. Gender-related differences in left ventricular chamber function. Cardiovascular Research. 2001;**49**:3-350. DOI: 10.1016/S0008-6363(00)00280-7

Chapter 5

Do Women Have a Higher Risk of Adverse Events after Carotid Revascularization?

Renato Casana, Chiara Malloggi,
Valerio Stefano Tolva, Andrea Odero Jr,
Richard Bulbulia, Alison Halliday,
Vincenzo Silani and Gianfranco Parati

Additional information is available at the end of the chapter

http://dx.doi.org/10.5772/intechopen.79527

Abstract

Carotid artery stenosis is thought to cause up to 10% of ischemic strokes. Till now, the optimal treatment between carotid endarterectomy (CEA) and carotid artery stenting (CAS) remains debated, in particular for specific subgroups of patients. Available data suggest that female have higher risk of perioperative adverse events, but conflicting results comparing CEA and CAS regarding the benefit for male or female are present in the literature. A systematic review of recent publications on gender-related differences in operative risks is reported. Moreover, a consecutive cohort of 912 symptomatic and asymptomatic patients undergoing CEA (407, 44.6%) or CAS (505, 55.4%) in a single institution has been evaluated to determine the influence of gender (59.7% male vs. 40.3% female) on the outcomes after both revascularization procedures at 30 days and during 3 years of follow-up. Our experience seems to confirm literature data as regarding female higher risk of restenosis. Female patients had higher periprocedural (2.7% female vs. 0.9% male; $p < 0.05$) and long-term (11.4% female vs. 4.6% male; $p < 0.05$) restenosis rate. In conclusion, female anatomic and pathologic parameters should be taken into account for an accurate diagnosis of carotid stenosis and guidelines should be adjusted consequently.

Keywords: carotid endarterectomy, complications, gender, mortality, restenosis, stenting

1. Introduction

Carotid artery stenting (CAS) might be a potentially safe and effective therapeutic alternative to carotid endarterectomy (CEA) for carotid artery disease, especially in high-risk patients, because CAS may avoid anesthetic and surgical risk. In this regard, the merit of using CAS has been questioned in specific subgroups of patients [1, 2]. The role of gender in the selection of the most effective carotid intervention remains a matter of debate. Historically, large randomized controlled studies looking at CEA had indicated an increased perioperative risk for women when gender subgroup analysis was performed. Additionally, all of the large CEA trials showed decreased or no benefit in women when compared to men mostly because these trials were underpowered to show any utility in the relatively small female population studied and, secondly, because the long-term benefit was undermined by the high perioperative morbidity seen in women [3, 4]. The SAPPHIRE trial was the first stenting trial to show noninferiority of CAS to CEA in high-risk patients, but the study did not compare outcomes for gender subgroups and women were underrepresented within the recruited population [5]. More recent trials reported conflicting results regarding risk of peri- and postprocedural adverse events for women and men [1, 6]. Then, reports comparing CEA and CAS failed either to analyze the influence of gender or to show a clear benefit for men or women [7].

Thus, to further inform the debate, we sought to conduct a systematic review of recent publications to assess epidemiologic and diagnostic hypotheses, which could underpin gender-related differences. Moreover, we report a retrospective observational study to determine the impact of gender on the outcomes of both carotid interventions in our institution.

2. Gender: stroke epidemiology and carotid disease

2.1. Gender differences in stroke epidemiology

An extensive review on gender differences in stroke epidemiology has shown that stroke is more common in men than in women and male patients are on average younger than female when they are affected by their first stroke [8]. Western European studies demonstrated that stroke incidence was about 30% higher in men than in women, but the strokes that did occur in women tended to be more severe [9]. During the last decade, an extensive number of papers have been published on epidemiological differences between genders.

A systematic review around gender differences in stroke epidemiology, presented by Appelros et al., including 59 incidence studies from 19 countries and 5 continents, showed that the mean age at first-ever stroke was 68.6 years among men and 72.9 years among women [10]. Stroke incidence and prevalence rates were 33 and 41% higher in male than in female, respectively, with large variations between age bands and between populations. The incidence rates of brain infarction and intracerebral hemorrhage were higher among men, whereas the rate of subarachnoid hemorrhage was higher among women, although this difference was not statistically significant. Stroke tended to be more severe in women with a 1-month case fatality of 24.7% compared with 19.7% for men.

The lower stroke incidence in women has been analyzed in systematic reviews in the last decades. A plausible reason might be the protective role of ovarian estrogen on the cerebral circulation [11–13], even if randomized trials currently recommend that postmenopausal hormone therapy should not be used in the primary prevention of stroke [14].

Other possible factors might be genetic factors, but no evidence for this expectation was found in the literature. Conversely, a recent systematic review showed that women with stroke have a higher familiarity of stroke than men [15].

Numerous studies have shown that blood pressure value was higher in men than women of same age [16, 17]. Moreover, peripheral artery disease [18, 19], ischemic heart disease [18, 20–22], and cigarette consumption [18–20, 23, 24] are more frequent among male stroke patients. Women have been shown to be at higher risk than men for atrial fibrillation-related cardioembolic stroke [22, 25–28]. The Swedish Stroke Register has shown that women with atrial fibrillation receive oral anticoagulant therapy less often than men [24]. The higher prevalence of embolic strokes among women could justify their higher stroke severity.

2.2. Diagnostic criteria for carotid stenosis by gender

The North American Symptomatic Carotid Endarterectomy Trial (NASCET) investigators standardized the method of quantifying the degree of carotid stenosis, and they considered arteriography the most predictable method for evaluating carotid stenosis [29].

Carotid duplex ultrasound scan (DUS) compares favorably with arteriography, and many physicians are using carotid DUS as the definitive diagnostic procedure before CEA even if it is mandatory to submit the patient to computer tomography angiography (CTA) or magnetic resonance angiography (MRA) for CAS to explore arch anatomy [30, 31]. Diagnostic criteria for carotid DUS have been accepted as predictable from laboratories accredited by the Intersocietal Commission for the Accreditation of Vascular Laboratories with ongoing quality programs.

Nevertheless, carotid DUS frequently resulted in overestimation of disease severity in women. This underlined the issue that women may have higher velocities in their carotid arteries than men for similar carotid stenosis. The question is: Are we overdiagnosing disease in women according to gender differences in carotid stenosis? The purpose of Comerota's study was to examine whether there were velocity differences based on gender in patients with carotid artery disease and whether different velocity criteria should be used in women, especially at clinically relevant thresholds of disease [32].

Patients who underwent carotid arteriography and carotid DUS were the basis for this study. Data from 1019 carotid bifurcations were available. Comparison was performed on the basis of 938 carotid arteries. Analyses were made in 536 male and 402 female carotid arteries. Arteriography was performed on average 23 days after the ultrasound examination, with 74% of arteriographic examinations performed within 30 days and 95% performed within 82 days of carotid DUS. Additionally, the single most diseased artery per patient was analyzed by gender. Peak systolic velocity (PSV) and end-diastolic velocity (EDV) were averaged for data subsets according to 10% intervals of internal carotid artery (ICA) stenoses. For all intervals, PSV and EDV averaged 9 and 6% higher in women than in men. Significant gender differences existed between PSV and EDV for 60 and 70% stenoses. For 70% stenosis, PSV averaged 285 $\pm$ 16 cm/s in women and

236 ± 11 cm/s in men ($p = 0.01$) and EDV averaged 79 ± 7 cm/s in women and 77 ± 6 cm/s in men ($p = 0.03$). For 60% stenosis, PSV averaged 228 ± 14 cm/s in women and 189 ± 11 cm/s in men ($p = 0.03$) and EDV averaged 68 ± 6 cm/s in women and 51 ± 4 cm/s in men ($p = 0.01$).

Williams et al. demonstrated that the diameter of the common carotid arteries (CCA), ICA, and external carotid arteries (ECA) were considerably smaller in women compared to those in men [33]. Schultz et al. showed a remarkable gender-specific difference in the distribution of atherosclerotic plaque. They reviewed 5395 arteriograms from the European Carotid Surgery Trial and compared diameter ratios of the ICA, CCA, and ECA with minimal disease to obtain a real relationship between vessels [34]. Among the 2930 arteriograms available for review, the mean ICA/CCA, ICA/ECA, and outflow/inflow area ratios were larger in women than in men ($p < 0.0001$). In addition, there were differences in the distribution of carotid plaque, with men more likely to have maximal stenosis in the ICA and women having a greater degree of plaque within the carotid bulb. Moreover, women appeared to have more severe disease in the ECA, which would also bias the distribution of existing flow velocity through the patent ICA.

Hansen et al. showed changes in arterial wall compliance in women who display higher age-related stiffness of their arteries and develop a higher degree of pulsatility with a higher velocity for any given blood pressure [35, 36].

Moreover, the natural history of carotid atherosclerosis emerges to be divergent in women compared with men. Independently from age, the risk for stroke is higher in men than in women [37]. The risk for stroke is greater in men with similar degrees of carotid stenosis [4, 29, 38] due to the fact that men have greater prevalence of high-risk carotid plaques. Joakimsen et al. showed that atherosclerotic lesions in men were more instable and ultrasound characteristics showed soft and lipid-rich plaques, with more common intraplaque hemorrhage. These characteristics are associated with an increased risk for ischemic events, including myocardial infarction (MI) and stroke [39–41].

According to those anatomic and pathologic gender-related differences, the higher velocity profiles observed in women compared with men could be explained. It needs to be adjusted in guidelines for an accurate and proper diagnosis in carotid stenosis in the near future.

2.2.1. Women gender-specific parameters

- Considerably smaller carotid diameter.
- Higher arterial velocity in carotid artery: PSV and EDV.
- Different distribution of atherosclerotic plaque with greater degree of plaque within the carotid bulb and more severe disease in the ECA.
- Different arterial wall compliance with higher age-related stiffness and higher degree of pulsatility.
- Presence of artifacts increasing arterial velocity (anemia).

3. Carotid revascularization: gender differences

3.1. Carotid revascularization outcomes in women compared with men

The literature shows that women have a higher risk of perioperative adverse events during carotid revascularization. In the Asymptomatic Carotid Atherosclerosis Study (ACAS), women had a higher rate of perioperative events (3.6% female [F] vs. 1.7% male [M]) during CEA [42] with a lower rate of events for female (8.7% F vs. 12.1% M) treated with best medical therapy. This result shows a lower 5-year risk reduction for female (17%) compared with male (66%).

The Asymptomatic Carotid Surgery Trial (ACST) suggested a lower long-term benefit of surgery for female, with male collecting a higher 5-year risk reduction than female (8.21% M vs. 4.08% F) [43]. In the International Carotid Stenting Study (ICSS), female had a higher 120-day event rate for CEA (7.6% F vs. 4.2% M) but a lower rate for CAS (8.0% F vs. 8.7% M) [44]. Reverse results was found in the Carotid Revascularization Endarterectomy vs. Stenting Trial (CREST) [6]. In this study, 2502 patients were randomly assigned to CEA (n = 1240) or CAS (n = 1262), 872 (34.9%) of whom were female. Rates of the primary endpoint for CAS compared with CEA were 6.2% vs. 6.8% in male (hazard ratio [HR] 0.99, 95% confidence interval [CI] 0.66–1.46) and 8.9% vs. 6.7% in female (HR 1.35, 95% CI 0.82–2.23). There was no significant interaction in the primary endpoint between genders (interaction $p = 0.34$). Periprocedural events occurred in 35 (4.3%) of 807 males assigned to CAS compared with 40 (4.9%) of 823 assigned to CEA (HR 0.90, 95% CI 0.57–1.41) and 31 (6.8%) of 455 females assigned to CAS compared with 16 (3.8%) of 417 assigned to CEA (HR 1.84, 95% CI 1.01–3.37; interaction $p = 0.064$).

In 2014, Jim et al. presented data from the Society for Vascular Surgery Vascular Registry to determine the effect of gender on outcomes after carotid revascularization [45]. There were 9865 patients (40.6% female) who underwent CEA (n = 6492) and CAS (n = 3373). The primary end point was a composite of death, stroke, and MI at 30 days. There were no differences in age and ethnicity between genders, but males were more likely to be symptomatic (41.6% M vs. 38.6% F; $p < 0.003$). There was a higher prevalence of hypertension and chronic obstructive pulmonary disease in female, whereas male had a higher prevalence of coronary artery disease, history of MI, and smoking history. For disease etiology in CAS, restenosis was more common in female (28.7% F vs. 19.7% M; $p < 0.0001$) and radiation was higher in male (6.2% M vs. 2.6% F; $p < 0.0001$). Comparing by gender, there were no statistically significant differences in the primary endpoint for CEA (4.07% F vs. 4.06% M) or CAS (6.69% F vs. 6.80% M). There were no differences after stratification by symptomatology and multivariate risk adjustment. These divergent results seem to be associated with different factors. In the last decades, best medical therapy improved significantly with a wide disposability of statins and antiplatelets with beneficial results on patient outcomes [46]. Another factor seems the fact that females were underrepresented in carotid randomized controlled trials [6].

4. Do women have a higher risk of adverse events after carotid revascularization in our experience?

4.1. Study design

A database of 912 consecutive patients with symptomatic or asymptomatic carotid artery stenosis undergoing CEA or CAS for carotid revascularization in the Department of Surgery of a single Institution from 2010 to 2017 was analyzed. Carotid stenosis was ≥80% for asymptomatic or ≥50% for symptomatic patients, as detected by DUS and confirmed by CTA or MRA using NASCET criteria [29].

The choice of revascularization technique (CAS/CEA) was based on general guideline recommendations, for example, European Society for Vascular Surgery (ESVS), American College of Cardiology and American Heart Association (ACC/AHA), and the team center experience according to morphologic and clinical data indicating best suitability with the aim of performing CAS and CEA with low procedural risks. Usually, patients with unfavorable aortic arch anatomy, severe peripheral vascular disease precluding femoral access, or extremely tortuous carotid anatomy were excluded from CAS. Similarly, unstable plaque, known allergies to aspirin, clopidogrel, or contrast media, and renal insufficiency (creatinine ≥1.5 mg/dL) were considered exclusion criteria for CAS.

4.2. CAS and CEA protocols

For CAS, the patient was given dual antiplatelet therapy beginning 1 day before the procedure. All patients received a 300 mg loading dose of clopidogrel 1 hour before the procedure.

Clinical investigation included a baseline assessment of a physical examination, carotid DUS of the supra-aortic vessels, procedural angiography, and neurological assessment measured using the National Institutes of Health Stroke Scale (NIHSS) [47]. All aortic arch types were included.

All procedures were performed following a standardized protocol in the operating room, equipped with a portable imaging fluoroscopic C-arm (OEC 9900 elite; GE Medical Siemens, Waukesha, WI, USA), by a single vascular team. Two skilled operators with high volume experience (>50 CEA/CAS procedures per year as first operator) performed all procedures [48–50]. Iodinated or gadolinium contrast was used in patients with normal creatinine level or creatinine >1.5 mg/dL (132 mmol/L), respectively. All patients received an intravenous heparin bolus (100 units/kg heparin) to achieve intraoperative anticoagulation (activated clotting time (ACT) ≥ 250 s throughout the procedure). In our center, with increasing experience, the number of CAS increased over time allowing CEA to be used for fewer and more complex cases in recent years. All procedures were carried out via femoral access. The introducer sheath (8 Fr) and guiding catheters (Zuma, Medtronic, MN, USA; Flexor, Cook Medical, IN, USA; Mach 1, Boston Scientific Corporation, MA, USA) ranged from 6 to 8 Fr, using inner catheters (coaxial method) with different shapes according to the anatomy of the arch (Imager II, Boston Scientific Corporation). Variable models of carotid stents (open-cell, closed-cell, hybrid, and micromesh stents) were employed, as a function of lesion characteristics and vessel anatomy. Temporary distal (Emboshield NAV6, Abbott Vascular, Santa Clara, CA, USA) or proximal (Mo.Ma, Medtronic, Minneapolis, MI, USA) cerebral protection devices were used as per internal protocol. Predilation was performed at the operator's discretion, with 2.0–4.0 mm TREK coronary balloons (Abbott Vascular). Postdilation was performed with a 4.5- or 5.5-mm diameter Rx Viatrac 14 Plus balloons (Abbott Vascular). CAS postoperative medical therapy included clopidogrel (75 mg once daily) for 1 month and aspirin (100 mg once daily) for a lifelong period.

For CEA, patients were usually maintained on aspirin therapy. CEA was performed under local anesthesia under electroencephalography (EEG) monitoring or transcutaneous oxygen saturation monitoring. Dacron or bovine pericardium graft angioplasty, or eversion endarterectomy were performed.

4.3. Procedural follow-up

Postprocedural patient evaluation was performed at the periprocedural (30 days) and at the postprocedural periods, at 3 months, 6 months, and yearly thereafter within 3 years, by a neurologist and a vascular surgeon.

Patient data were captured using a paper case report form. Symptoms status and exact information about clinical adverse events were obtained. Carotid DUS of the supra-aortic vessels was obtained to determine the degree of carotid stenosis.

4.4. Endpoints, definitions, and statistical analysis

Primary endpoints were rates of death; stroke; MI; a composite of the incidence of any stroke, MI, or death; and restenosis within 30 days. Secondary endpoints were rates of death; stroke; MI; a composite of the incidence of any stroke, MI, or death; and restenosis, during the follow-up period, within 36 months after the procedure.

For the composite of any stroke, MI, or death, patients might have had more than one event. For example, fatal stroke events are included in both death and stroke outcomes, and subjects might have had both an ipsilateral and a subsequent contralateral stroke. The diagnosis and quantification of restenosis was performed using carotid DUS. Carotid restenosis was set at ≥40% [51, 52].

Categorical variables were reported as number and percentages. For numeric variables, minimum, maximum, mean, and standard deviation were calculated. Continuous data are presented as percentages or mean ± standard deviation (SD). Rates for comorbidities, complications, and 30-day outcomes were compared between male and female patients and between those undergoing CAS and CEA by χ^2 test. Survival, stroke, MI, and restenosis rates were calculated using Kaplan-Meier analysis to compensate for patient dropouts and were reported using current Society for Vascular Surgery (SVS) criteria [53]. Standard errors (SE) are reported in Kaplan-Meier analyses. The log-rank test was used to determine differences among patients submitted to CEA and CAS.

A value of $p < 0.05$ was considered statistically significant for all measurements. All analyses were performed using STATA™ (STATA Corp., version 14.0, College Station, TX, USA).

The study was approved by the local Ethic Committee of Istituto Auxologico Italiano (statement CE 30.05.2006). Written consent was obtained from all patients before both CAS and CEA revascularization.

4.5. Results

From 2010 to 2017, a total of 912 patients underwent interventions for carotid stenosis. There were 544 (59.7%) males and 368 (40.3%) females. Mean age was 71.1 ± 8.6 and 69.4 ± 9.0 for male and female patients, respectively. About 193 (35.4%) male and 128 (34.7%) female patients were symptomatic. Of the 912 carotid revascularizations, 407 (44.6%) were by CEA and 505 (55.4%) were by CAS. Demographic and baseline characteristics of study participants after separation by gender and procedure are presented in **Table 1**. Female patients were older (72.1 ± 9.0 F vs. 68.4 ± 8.6 M, $p < 0.05$) and more likely to have a history of hypertension (79.7% F vs. 72.5% M, $p < 0.05$) and hyperlipidemia (74.4% F vs. 69.2% M, $p < 0.05$) with respect to male patients. Male patients were more likely to be smokers (35.0% M vs. 33.3% F, $p < 0.05$) and to have history of MI (19.7% M vs. 17.5% F, $p < 0.05$), chronic renal insufficiency (20.5% M vs. 11.9% F, $p < 0.05$), and CAD (28.0% M vs. 26.1% F, $p < 0.05$). The distribution of comorbidities within the two procedural groups was similar. For CAS patients, men were more likely to have diabetes (37.9% M vs. 33.5% F, $p < 0.05$) and chronic renal insufficiency (18.0% M vs. 13.8% F, $p < 0.05$) and women had a higher prevalence of hypertension (89.5% F vs. 71.5% M, $p < 0.05$) and hyperlipidemia (82.9% F vs. 72.0% M, $p < 0.05$). For CEA patients, men tended to have a higher prevalence of history of MI (20.3% M vs. 16.0% F, $p < 0.05$) and chronic renal

	M (n = 544)	F (n = 368)	CEA (n = 407)		CAS (n = 505)	
			M (n = 326)	F (n = 200)	M (n = 241)	F (n = 145)
Age, mean ± SD	68.4 ± 8.6	72.1 ± 9.0	68.9 ± 8.5	71.5 ± 9.3	68.0 ± 8.7	72.8 ± 8.6
Symptomatic, n (%)	193 (35.4%)	128 (34.7%)	108 (33.1%)	70 (34.9%)	85 (35.0%)	58 (40.1%)
Smokers, n (%)	191 (35.0%)	123 (33.3%)	109 (33.4%)	77 (38.8%)	82 (33.8%)	45 (31.3%)
Hypertension, n (%)	395 (72.5%)	293 (79.7%)	222 (68.0%)	164 (82.0%)	173 (71.5%)	129 (89.5%)
Diabetes, n (%)	172 (31.7%)	127 (34.5%)	81 (24.8%)	78 (39.3%)	91 (37.9%)	48 (33.5%)
Hyperlipidemia, n (%)	376 (69.2%)	274 (74.4%)	202 (62.0%)	154 (77.1%)	174 (72.0%)	120 (82.9%)
CAD, n (%)	152 (28.0%)	96 (26.1%)	86 (26.4%)	55 (27.5%)	66 (27.3%)	41 (28.5%)
History of stroke, n (%)	133 (24.5%)	78 (21.3%)	71 (21.9%)	44 (21.8%)	62 (25.6%)	35 (24.0%)
History of MI, n (%)	107 (19.7%)	64 (17.5%)	66 (20.3%)	32 (16.0%)	41 (17.0%)	32 (22.4%)
Chronic renal insufficiency, n (%)	112 (20.5%)	44 (11.9%)	68 (20.9%)	24 (12.0%)	43 (18.0%)	20 (13.8%)
CHF, n (%)	54 (9.8%)	42 (11.5%)	29 (8.8%)	19 (9.5%)	25 (10.3%)	23 (16.1%)
COPD, n (%)	105 (19.4%)	54 (14.6%)	61 (18.6%)	30 (15.1%)	45 (18.5%)	24 (16.5%)
Cancer history, n (%)	101 (18.6%)	72 (19.5%)	53 (16.3%)	37 (18.5%)	48 (19.7%)	35 (24.1%)

M: male; F: female; CEA: carotid endarterectomy; CAS: carotid artery stenting; SD: standard deviation; CAD: coronary artery disease; MI: myocardial infarction; CHF: congestive heart failure; and COPD: chronic obstructive pulmonary disease.

Table 1. Baseline characteristics of study participants (n = 912).

insufficiency (20.9% M vs. 12.0% F, $p < 0.05$), whereas women had a higher prevalence of hypertension (82.0% F vs. 68.0% M, $p < 0.05$), diabetes (39.3% F vs. 24.8% M, $p < 0.05$), and hyperlipidemia (77.1% F vs. 62.0% M, $p < 0.05$).

Patients were required to undergo DUS and neurological examination at 1 month and subsequently at 3, 6, 12, 24, and 36 months after the procedure.

Periprocedural outcome measures in male patients compared with female patients are reported in **Table 2**. The death rate in the overall population was 0.3% (3/912), with no significant differences in rates between the two groups (0.4% M vs. 0.3% F) and between the two procedures (0.5% CEA vs. 0.2% CAS). Periprocedural outcomes were similar for male and female patients for 30-day death, stroke, MI, and a composite of any stroke, MI, or death rates. Female patients had higher periprocedural restenosis rate (2.7% F vs. 0.9% M; $p < 0.05$). Periprocedural outcomes were similar for CEA and CAS for 30-day death, stroke, and MI rates. Female patients undergoing CEA had a higher 30-day rate of any stroke, MI, or death (5.5% F vs. 3.1% M, $p < 0.05$). Female patients undergoing CAS had a higher 30-day rate of any stroke, MI, or death (7.6% F vs. 5.4% M, $p < 0.05$) and restenosis (4.8% F vs. 1.2% M, $p < 0.05$).

For long-term follow-up, 95, 91, 78, 75, and 62% of patients attended their 3-, 6-, 12-, 24-, and 36-month follow-up appointments, respectively. Patients were not able to attend follow-up mainly because they moved to remote locations or because they declined further visits for personal reasons. Most recent patients could not attend their 24- and 36-month appointments yet.

Long-term outcomes were similar for male and female patients for 36-month death and stroke. Male patients experienced a slightly higher rate of MI. Female patients had higher long-term restenosis rate (11.4% F vs. 4.6% M; $p < 0.05$). Female patients undergoing CEA had a higher 36-month rate of stroke (14.0% F vs. 6.7% M; $p < 0.05$) and restenosis (11.5% F vs. 2.5% M,

	M (n = 544)	F (n = 368)	CEA (n = 407)		CAS (n = 505)	
			M (n = 326)	F (n = 200)	M (n = 241)	F (n = 145)
Short-term (≤30 days) outcomes, n (%)						
Death	2 (0.4%)	1 (0.3%)	1 (0.3%)	1 (0.5%)	1 (0.4%)	0 (0.0%)
Stroke	7 (1.3%)	5 (1.4%)	2 (0.6%)	3 (1.5%)	5 (2.1%)	2 (1.4%)
MI	13 (2.4%)	10 (2.7%)	6 (1.8%)	5 (2.5%)	7 (2.9%)	5 (3.5%)
Stroke, MI, or death	9 (1.7%)	6 (1.6%)	10 (3.1%)	11 (5.5%)	13 (5.4%)	11 (7.6%)
Restenosis	5 (0.9%)	10 (2.7%)	2 (0.6%)	3 (1.5%)	3 (1.2%)	7 (4.8%)
Long-term (>30 days) outcomes, n (%)						
Death	37 (6.8%)	35 (9.5%)	17 (5.2%)	12 (6.0%)	20 (8.3%)	23 (15.9%)
Stroke	52 (9.6%)	59 (16.0%)	22 (6.7%)	28 (14.0%)	30 (12.4%)	31 (21.4%)
MI	38 (7.0%)	22 (6.0%)	20 (5.1%)	11 (4.1%)	18 (6.4%)	11 (5.2%)
Stroke, MI, or death	101 (18.6%)	87 (23.7%)	45 (13.8%)	46 (23.1%)	56 (23.2%)	41 (28.4%)
Restenosis	25 (4.6%)	42 (11.4%)	8 (2.5%)	23 (11.5%)	17 (7.0%)	19 (13.1%)

M: male; F: female; CEA: carotid endarterectomy; CAS: carotid angioplasty and stenting; and MI: myocardial infarction.

Table 2. Periprocedural (30 days) outcomes after carotid revascularization in male and female patients receiving CEA or CAS.

$p < 0.05$). No significant differences in long-term outcomes were observed between male and female patients undergoing CAS (**Table 2**).

The 36-month risk of any cause mortality was 5.6 (1.6)% (mean (SD)) for male patients and 15.2 (3.3)% for female patients, with a significant difference in Kaplan-Meier estimates at 36 months between the two groups according to log-rank test. Female patients undergoing CAS experience lower 3-year freedom from death rate, with no significance difference with respect to the other groups (82.5% vs. 94.5, 94.2, and 86.4% for F-CAS, M-CAS, M-CEA, and F-CEA patients, respectively, $p > 0.05$; **Figure 1**).

The risk of stroke at 36 months was 10.8 (2.2)% for male and 21.4 (3.7)% for female ($p < 0.05$). Male patients undergoing CEA had a higher 36-month freedom from stroke rate as compared to the other groups (91.6% vs. 85.8, 82.2, and 73.7% for M-CEA, M-CAS, F-CEA, and F-CAS patients, respectively, $p < 0.05$) with a significant difference in the comparison between M-CEA and F-CAS (**Figure 2**).

Male patients had a greater risk of MI than female patients. The 12-, 24-, and 36-month estimates of MI rates were 4.9 (1.4)%, 6.0 (1.6)%, and 7.6 (1.8)% for male and a constant rate equal to 5.8 (2.0)% for female ($p > 0.05$). There were no differences in the risk of experiencing a MI during follow-up among male and female patients undergoing CEA or CAS (**Figure 3**).

The overall risk of any stroke, MI, or death was equal to 20.4 (2.8)% for male patients and 30.9 (4.2)% for female patients ($p < 0.05$). The 3-year freedom from any stroke, MI, or death was 84.4, 72.6, 72.2, and 64.9% for M-CEA, M-CAS, F-CEA, and F-CAS patients, respectively, with significant differences in the comparison between M-CEA and F-CAS (**Figure 4**).

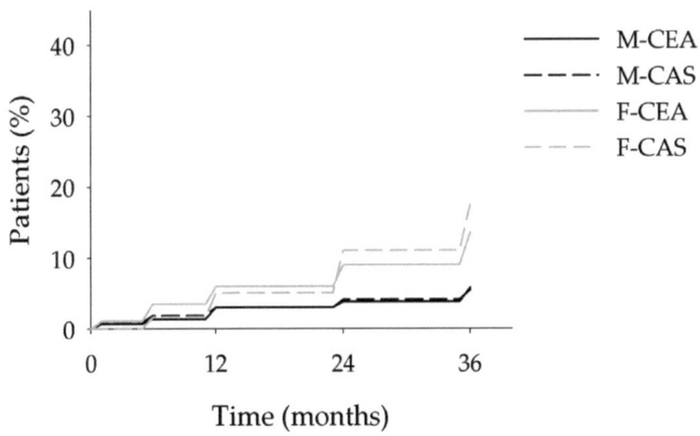

Months	0	1	3	6	12	24	36
M-CEA	326	326	326	308	292	244	230
M-CAS	241	241	241	228	217	182	171
F-CEA	200	200	200	189	176	146	135
F-CAS	145	145	145	139	130	107	96

Figure 1. Mortality. Male and female patients submitted to CEA or CAS who survived during follow-up. Error bars are omitted for clarity. Standard errors did not exceed 10% at all-time intervals that were analyzed. The number of patients at risk at each time interval is shown below the figure.

http://dx.doi.org/10.5772/intechopen.79527

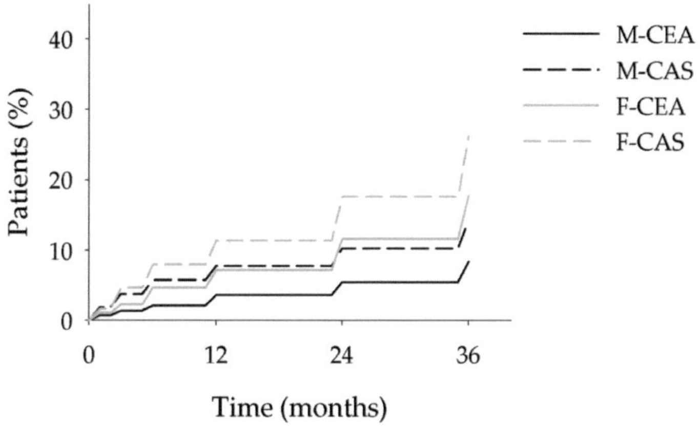

Months	0	1	3	6	12	24	36
M-CEA	326	326	324	306	290	242	226
M-CAS	241	241	236	221	207	171	157
F-CEA	200	200	197	187	173	144	130
F-CAS	145	145	143	132	121	98	87

Figure 2. Stroke. Male and female patients submitted to CEA or CAS who experienced a stroke during follow-up. Error bars are omitted for clarity. Standard errors did not exceed 10% at all-time intervals that were analyzed. The number of patients at risk at each time interval is shown below the figure.

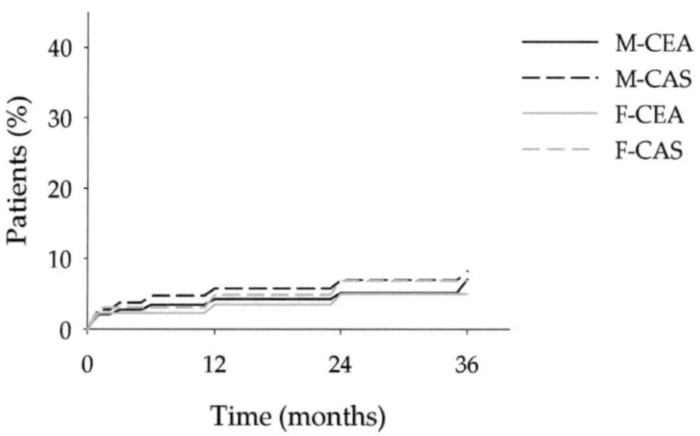

Months	0	1	3	6	12	24	36
M-CEA	326	326	319	301	285	239	226
M-CAS	241	241	234	221	210	176	164
F-CEA	200	200	200	201	178	150	150
F-CAS	145	145	145	146	128	107	107

Figure 3. Myocardial infarction (MI). Male and female patients submitted to CEA or CAS who experienced a MI during follow-up. Error bars are omitted for clarity. Standard errors did not exceed 10% at all-time intervals that were analyzed. The number of patients at risk at each time interval is shown below the figure.

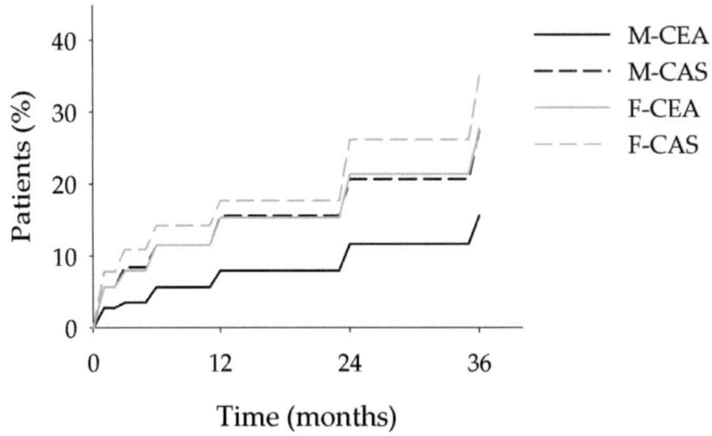

Months	0	1	3	6	12	24	36
M-CEA	326	326	317	299	278	228	207
M-CAS	241	241	228	210	194	153	135
F-CEA	200	200	189	176	160	128	112
F-CAS	145	145	135	123	112	89	75

Figure 4. Stroke, MI, or death. Male and female patients submitted to CEA or CAS who experienced any stroke, MI, or death during follow-up. Error bars are omitted for clarity. Standard errors did not exceed 10% at all-time intervals that were analyzed. The number of patients at risk at each time interval is shown below the figure.

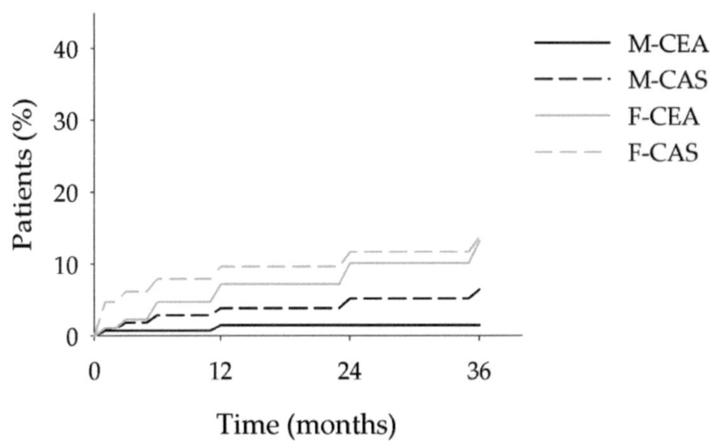

Months	0	1	3	6	12	24	36
M-CEA	326	326	326	326	294	294	294
M-CAS	241	238	237	223	212	178	166
F-CEA	200	200	198	187	173	144	132
F-CAS	145	145	139	130	121	100	93

Figure 5. Restenosis. Male and female patients submitted to CEA or CAS who experienced a restenosis during follow-up. Error bars are omitted for clarity. Standard errors did not exceed 10% at all-time intervals that were analyzed. The number of patients at risk at each time interval is shown below the figure.

During follow-up, female patients exhibited higher restenosis risk with respect to male [2.5 (1.0)%, 3.0 (1.1)%, and 3.6 (1.3)% vs. 8.2 (2.3)%, 10.8 (2.7)%, and 13.5 (3.0)% for 12-, 24-, and 36-month rates, for male and female patients, respectively ($p < 0.05$)]. Male patients undergoing CEA experienced higher freedom from restenosis rates at 3 years (98.5% vs. 93.5%, 86.8%, and 86.2%, for M-CEA, M-CAS, F-CEA, and F-CAS patients, respectively) with significant differences in the comparisons between M-CEA and F-CAS and between M-CEA and F-CEA (**Figure 5**).

5. Conclusion

Stroke has been shown to be more common in male than in female. Male patients are affected by first stroke on average in younger age with respect to female [8]. Stroke incidence was demonstrated to be about 30% higher in men than in women in Western European studies, but strokes in women tend to be more severe [9].

During the last decade, an extensive number of papers have been published on epidemiological differences between gender. The lower stroke incidence in female has been analyzed in systematic reviews in the last decades. Plausible reasons might be the protective role of ovarian estrogen on the cerebral circulation [11–13], genetic factors [15], sensitivity for antiplatelet therapy [54], lower blood pressure values [16, 17], lower frequency of peripheral artery diseases [18, 19], ischemic heart diseases [20–22], and cigarettes consumption [23, 24] in female patients with respect to male patients.

Carotid revascularization outcomes in female compared with male showed that the former have a higher risk of perioperative adverse events [55]. The ACAS reported a higher rate of perioperative events for female with respect to male (3.6% F vs. 1.7% M) during CEA [42] with a lower rate of events for female (8.7% F vs. 12.1% M) treated with best medical therapy. Moreover, this study showed a lower 5-year risk reduction for female (17% F vs. 66% M). In more recent trials, carotid revascularization outcomes were similar between genders, but restenosis was more common in female [6, 45].

In the study presented herein, 912 consecutive patients with symptomatic and asymptomatic carotid artery stenosis underwent CEA (44.6%) or CAS (55.4%) in a single institution. The death rate in the overall population was 0.3% (3/912), with no significant differences in rates between male and female patients (0.4% M vs. 0.3% F) and between the two procedures (0.5% CEA vs. 0.2% CAS).

Periprocedural outcomes were similar for male and female patients for 30-day death, stroke, MI, and a composite of any stroke, MI, or death rates. Female patients had higher periprocedural restenosis rate (2.7% F vs. 0.9% M; $p < 0.05$). Periprocedural outcomes were similar for CEA and CAS for 30-day death, stroke, and MI rates.

Female patients undergoing CEA had a higher 30-day rate of any stroke, MI, or death (5.5% F vs. 3.1% M, $p < 0.05$). Female patients undergoing CAS had also a higher 30-day risk of restenosis (4.8% F vs. 1.2% M, $p < 0.05$).

Long-term outcomes were similar for male and female patients for 36-month death and stroke. Female patients had higher long-term restenosis rate (11.4% F vs. 4.6% M; $p < 0.05$). Female patients undergoing CEA had a higher 36-month rate of stroke (14.0% F vs. 6.7% M; $p < 0.05$) and restenosis (11.5% F vs. 2.5% M, $p < 0.05$). No significant differences in long-term outcomes were observed between male and female patients undergoing CAS. Our monocentric experience seems to confirm literature data as regarding female higher risk of restenosis during CEA. These gender-associated differences should be taken into account for the treatment of carotid artery disease.

In light of this, in the near future, female anatomic and pathologic parameters should be used, such as carotid diameter which is considerably smaller in female than in male, thus determining higher arterial velocity in carotid artery. The greater degree of atherosclerotic plaque within the carotid bulb, the higher age-related arterial wall stiffness and degree of pulsatility, and the presence of artifacts increasing arterial velocity should be taken into account for an accurate diagnosis of carotid stenosis and guidelines should be adjusted consequently.

Gender subgroup analyses from large randomized trials, such as ACST-2, an international randomized trial comparing CEA with CAS for long-term stroke prevention, which planned the recruitment of 3600 patients by the end of 2019 [56–58], may report interesting and important results on the impact of gender on the peri- and postprocedural outcomes after carotid revascularization procedures.

Author details

Renato Casana[1,2]*, Chiara Malloggi[2], Valerio Stefano Tolva[3], Andrea Odero Jr[1], Richard Bulbulia[4], Alison Halliday[5], Vincenzo Silani[6,7] and Gianfranco Parati[8,9]

*Address all correspondence to: r.casana@auxologico.it

1 Department of Surgery, IRCCS Istituto Auxologico Italiano, Milan, Italy

2 Vascular Surgery Research Experimental Laboratory, IRCCS Istituto Auxologico Italiano, Milan, Italy

3 Department of Vascular Surgery, Policlinico Di Monza Hospital, Monza, Italy

4 Clinical Trial Service Unit, Nuffield Department of Population Health, University of Oxford, Oxford, UK

5 Nuffield Department of Surgical Sciences, University of Oxford, Oxford, UK

6 Department of Neurology-Stroke Unit and Laboratory of Neuroscience, IRCCS Istituto Auxologico Italiano, Milan, Italy

7 'Dino Ferrari' Centre, Department of Pathophysiology and Transplantation, Università degli Studi di Milano, Milan, Italy

8 Department of Cardiology, IRCCS Istituto Auxologico Italiano, Milan, Italy

9 Department of Health Sciences, Università degli Studi di Milano-Bicocca, Milan, Italy

References

[1] Carotid Stenting Trialists' Collaboration, Bonati LH, Dobson J, Algra A, Branchereau A, Chatellier G, et al. Short-term outcome after stenting versus endarterectomy for symptomatic carotid stenosis: A preplanned meta-analysis of individual patient data. Lancet. 2010;**376**:1062-1073. DOI: 10.1016/S0140-6736(10)61009-4

[2] Eckstein H-H, Ringleb P, Allenberg J-R, Berger J, Fraedrich G, Hacke W, et al. Results of the stent-protected angioplasty versus carotid endarterectomy (SPACE) study to treat symptomatic stenoses at 2 years: A multinational, prospective, randomised trial. Lancet Neurology. 2008;**7**:893-902. DOI: 10.1016/S1474-4422(08)70196-0

[3] Collaborators NASCET. Beneficial effect of carotid endarterectomy in symptomatic patients with high-grade carotid stenosis. The New England Journal of Medicine. 1991; **325**:445-453. DOI: 10.1056/NEJM199108153250701

[4] European Carotid Surgery Trialists' Collaborative Group. MRC European carotid surgery trial: Interim results for symptomatic patients with severe (70–99%) or with mild (0–29%) carotid stenosis. Lancet. 1991;**337**:1235-1243. DOI: 10.1016/0140-6736(91)92916-P

[5] Yadav J, Wholey M, Kuntz R, Fayad P, Katzen B, Mishkel G, et al. Protected carotid artery stenting versus endaerterectomy in high risk patients. The New England Journal of Medicine. 2004;**351**:1493-1501. DOI: 10.1056/NEJMoa1208410

[6] Howard VJ, Lutsep HL, Mackey A, Demaerschalk BM, Sam AD, Gonzales NR, et al. Influence of sex on outcomes of stenting versus endarterectomy: A subgroup analysis of the carotid revascularization endarterectomy versus stenting trial (CREST). Lancet Neurology. 2011;**10**:530-537. DOI: 10.1016/S1474-4422(11)70080-1

[7] Goldstein LJ, Khan HU, Sambol EB, Kent KC, Faries PL, Vouyouka AG. Carotid artery stenting is safe and associated with comparable outcomes in men and women. Journal of Vascular Surgery. 2009;**49**:315-324. DOI: 10.1016/j.jvs.2008.08.110

[8] Wyller TB. Stroke and gender. The Journal of Gender-Specific Medicine. 1999;**2**:41-45

[9] Sudlow CL, Warlow CP. Comparing stroke incidence worldwide: What makes studies comparable? Stroke. 1996;**27**:550-558

[10] Appelros P, Stegmayr B, Terent A. Sex differences in stroke epidemiology: A systematic review. Stroke. 2009;**40**:1082-1090. DOI: 10.1161/STROKEAHA.108.540781

[11] Murphy SJ, McCullough LD, Smith JM. Stroke in the female: Role of biological sex and estrogen. ILAR Journal. 2004;**45**:147-159

[12] Krause DN, Duckles SP, Pelligrino DA. Influence of sex steroid hormones on cerebrovascular function. Journal of Applied Physiology. 2006;**101**:1252-1261. DOI: 10.1152/japplphysiol.01095.2005

[13] Alonso de Leciñana M, Egido JA, Fernández C, Martínez-Vila E, Santos S, Morales A, et al. Risk of ischemic stroke and lifetime estrogen exposure. Neurology. 2007;**68**:33-38. DOI: 10.1212/01.wnl.0000250238.69938.f5

[14] Goldstein LB, Adams R, Alberts MJ, Appel LJ, Brass LM, Bushnell CD, et al. Primary prevention of ischemic stroke: A guideline from the American Heart Association/American Stroke Association Stroke Council: Cosponsored by the Atherosclerotic Peripheral Vascular Disease Interdisciplinary Working Group; Cardiovascular Nursing Council. Stroke. 2006;**37**:1583-1633. DOI: 10.1161/01.STR.0000223048.70103.F1

[15] Touze E, Rothwell PM. Sex differences in heritability of ischemic stroke: A systematic review and meta-analysis. Stroke. 2008;**39**:16-23. DOI: 10.1161/STROKEAHA.107.484618

[16] Khoury S, Yarows SA, O'Brien TK, Sowers JR. Ambulatory blood pressure monitoring in a nonacademic setting. Effects of age and sex. American Journal of Hypertension. 1992;**5**: 616-623

[17] Wiinberg N, Høegholm A, Christensen HR, Bang LE, Mikkelsen KL, Nielsen PE, et al. 24-h ambulatory blood pressure in 352 normal Danish subjects, related to age and gender. American Journal of Hypertension. 1995;**8**:978-986. DOI: 10.1016/0895-7061(95)00216-2

[18] Arboix A, Oliveres M, García-Eroles L, Maragall C, Massons J, Targa C. Acute cerebrovascular disease in women. European Neurology. 2001;**45**:199-205. DOI: 10.1159/000052130

[19] Roquer J, Campello AR, Gomis M. Sex differences in first-ever acute stroke. Stroke. 2003; **34**:1581-1585. DOI: 10.1161/01.STR.0000078562.82918.F6

[20] Jorgensen HS, Weber U, Nakayama H, Kammersgaard LP, Olsen TS. Differences in risk factor distribution, initial stroke severity, and outcome in men and women. The Copenhagen Stroke Study. Cerebrovascular Diseases. 1999;**9**(Suppl 1):9-19

[21] Holroyd-Leduc JM, Kapral MK, Austin PC, Tu JV. Sex differences and similarities in the management and outcome of stroke patients. Stroke. 2000;**31**:1833-1837

[22] Fang MC, Singer DE, Chang Y, Hylek EM, Henault LE, Jensvold NG, et al. Gender differences in the risk of ischemic stroke and peripheral embolism in atrial fibrillation: The AnTicoagulation and Risk Factors in Atrial Fibrillation (ATRIA) Study. Circulation. 2005;**112**:1687-1691. DOI: 10.1161/CIRCULATIONAHA.105.553438

[23] Worrall BB, Johnston KC, Kongable G, Hung E, Richardson D, Gorelick PB. Stroke risk factor profiles in African American women: An interim report from the African-American Antiplatelet Stroke Prevention Study. Stroke. 2002;**33**:913-919

[24] Glader E-L, Stegmayr B, Norrving B, Terént A, Hulter-Asberg K, Wester P-O, et al. Sex differences in management and outcome after stroke: A Swedish national perspective. Stroke. 2003;**34**:1970-1975. DOI: 10.1161/01.STR.0000083534.81284.C5

[25] Stroke Prevention in Atrial Fibrillation Investigators. Risk factors for thromboembolism during aspirin therapy in patients with atrial fibrillation: The stroke prevention in atrial

fibrillation study. Journal of Stroke and Cerebrovascular Diseases. 1995;**5**:147-157. DOI: 10.1016/S1052-3057(10)80166-1

[26] Stewart S, Hart CL, Hole DJ, McMurray JJV. A population-based study of the long-term risks associated with atrial fibrillation: 20-year follow-up of the Renfrew/Paisley study. The American Journal of Medicine. 2002;**113**:359-364

[27] Wang TJ, Massaro JM, Levy D, Vasan RS, Wolf PA, D'Agostino RB, et al. A risk score for predicting stroke or death in individuals with new-onset atrial fibrillation in the community. Journal of American Medical Association. 2003;**290**:1049. DOI: 10.1001/jama.290.8.1049

[28] Friberg J, Scharling H, Gadsbøll N, Truelsen T, Jensen GB, Copenhagen City Heart Study. Comparison of the impact of atrial fibrillation on the risk of stroke and cardiovascular death in women versus men (The Copenhagen City Heart Study). The American Journal of Cardiology. 2004;**94**:889-894. DOI: 10.1016/j.amjcard.2004.06.023

[29] Collaborators NASCET. Beneficial effects of carotid endarterectomy in symptomatic patients with high-grade carotid stenosis. The New England Journal of Medicine. 1991; **325**:445-453

[30] Flanigan DP, Schuler JJ, Vogel M, Borozan PG, Gray B, Sobinsky KR. The role of carotid duplex scanning in surgical decision making. Journal of Vascular Surgery. 1985;**2**:15-25. DOI: 10.1016/0741-5214(85)90171-5

[31] Zwolak RM. Carotid endarterectomy without angiography: Are we ready? Vascular Surgery. 1997;**31**:1-9. DOI: 10.1177/153857449703100101

[32] Comerota AJ. Gender differences in carotid stenosis: Are we overdiagnosing disease in women? Vascular. 2006

[33] Ford CS, Howard VJ, Howard G, Frye JL, Toole JF, McKinney WM. The sex difference in manifestations of carotid bifurcation disease. Stroke. 1986;**17**:877-881. DOI: 10.1161/01.STR.17.5.877

[34] Scheel P, Ruge C, Schöning M. Flow velocity and flow volume measurements in the extracranial carotid and vertebral arteries in healthy adults: Reference data and the effects of age. Ultrasound in Medicine & Biology. 2000;**26**:1261-1266. DOI: 10.1016/S0301-5629(00)00293-3

[35] Schulz UG, Rothwell PM. Sex differences in carotid bifurcation anatomy and the distribution of atherosclerotic plaque. Stroke. 2001;**32**:1525-1531

[36] Hansen F, Mangell P, Sonesson B, Länne T. Diameter and compliance in the human common carotid artery—variations with age and sex. Ultrasound in Medicine & Biology. 1995;**21**:1-9

[37] Brass LM, Pavlakis SG, DeVivo D, Piomelli S, Mohr JP. Transcranial Doppler measurements of the middle cerebral artery. Effect of hematocrit. Stroke. 1988;**19**:1466-1469. DOI: 10.1161/01.STR.19.12.1466

[38] Barnett HJM, Taylor DW, Eliasziw M, Fox AJ, Ferguson GG, Haynes RB, et al. Benefit of carotid endarterectomy in patients with symptomatic moderate or severe stenosis. The New England Journal of Medicine. 1998;**339**:1415-1425. DOI: 10.1056/NEJM199811123392002

[39] Barnett HJM, Meldrum HE, Eliasziw M, North American Symptomatic Carotid Endarterectomy Trial (NASCET) collaborators. The appropriate use of carotid endarterectomy. Canadian Medical Association Journal. 2002;**166**:1169-1179

[40] Joakimsen O, Bonaa KH, Stensland-Bugge E, Jacobsen BK. Age and sex differences in the distribution and ultrasound morphology of carotid atherosclerosis: The Tromsø Study. Arteriosclerosis, Thrombosis, and Vascular Biology. 1999;**19**:3007-3013. DOI: 10.1161/01.ATV.19.12.3007

[41] Fuster V. Elucidation of the role of plaque instability and rupture in acute coronary events. The American Journal of Cardiology. 1995;**76**:24C-33C

[42] Executive Committee for the Asymptomatic Carotid Atherosclerosis Study. Endarterectomy for asymptomatic carotid artery stenosis. Journal of American Medical Association. 1995;**273**:1421-1428

[43] Halliday A, Mansfield A, Marro J, Peto C, Peto R, Potter J, et al. Prevention of disabling and fatal strokes by successful carotid endarterectomy in patients without recent neurological symptoms: Randomised controlled trial. Lancet. 2004;**363**:1491-1502. DOI: 10.1016/S0140-6736(04)16146-1

[44] International Carotid Stenting Study investigators, Ederle J, Dobson J, Featherstone RL, Bonati LH, van der Worp HB, et al. Carotid artery stenting compared with endarterectomy in patients with symptomatic carotid stenosis (International Carotid Stenting Study): An interim analysis of a randomised controlled trial. Lancet (London, England). 2010;**375**:985-997. DOI: 10.1016/S0140-6736(10)60239-5

[45] Jim J, Dillavou ED, Upchurch GR, Osborne NH, Kenwood CT, Siami FS, et al. Gender-specific 30-day outcomes after carotid endarterectomy and carotid artery stenting in the Society for Vascular Surgery Vascular Registry. Journal of Vascular Surgery. 2014;**59**:742-748. DOI: 10.1016/J.JVS.2013.09.036

[46] National Cholesterol Education Program (NCEP). Expert panel on detection, evaluation, and treatment of high blood cholesterol in adults (adult treatment panel III). Third report of the national cholesterol education program (NCEP) expert panel on detection, evaluation, and treatment of high blood cholesterol in adults (adult treatment panel III) final report. Circulation. 2002;**106**:3143-3421

[47] Lyden P, Brott T, Tilley B, Welch KM, Mascha EJ, Levine S, et al. Improved reliability of the NIH stroke scale using video training. NINDS TPA Stroke Study Group. Stroke. 1994;**25**:2220-2226. DOI: 10.1161/01.STR.25.11.2220

[48] Casana R, Tolva V, Odero A Jr, Malloggi C, Paolucci A, Triulzi F, et al. Safety and efficacy of the new micromesh-covered stent CGuard in patients undergoing carotid artery

stenting: Early experience from a single Centre. European Journal of Vascular and Endovascular Surgery. 2017;**54**:681-687. DOI: 10.1016/J.EJVS.2017.09.015

[49] Casana R, Halliday A, Bianchi P, Fresa E, Silani V, Parati G, et al. Carotid artery stenting in patients with acute coronary syndrome: A possible primary therapy for symptomatic carotid stenosis. Journal of Endovascular Therapy. 2013;**20**:546-551. DOI: 10.1583/13-4244.1

[50] Tolva V, Bertoni GB, Bianchi PG, Keller GC, Casana R. Immediate surgery for acute internal carotid artery dissection and thrombosis during filter deployment prior to stenting: A case report. Vascular. 2013;**21**:247-250. DOI: 10.1177/1708538113478774

[51] Parlani G, De Rango P, Cieri E, Verzini F, Giordano G, Simonte G, et al. Diabetes is not a predictor of outcome for carotid revascularization with stenting as it may be for carotid endarterectomy. Journal of Vascular Surgery. 2012;**55**:79-89. DOI: 10.1016/j.jvs.2011.07.080

[52] Faught WE, Mattos M, van Bemmelen PS, Hodgson KJ, Barkmeier LD, Ramsey DE, et al. Color-flow duplex scanning of carotid arteries: New velocity criteria based on receiver operator characteristic analysis for threshold stenoses used in the symptomatic and asymptomatic carotid trials. Journal of Vascular Surgery. 1994;**19**:818-828. DOI: 10.1016/S0741-5214(94)70006-0

[53] Baker JD, Rutherford RB, Bernstein EF, Courbier R, Ernst CB, Kempczinski RF, et al. Suggested standards for reports dealing with cerebrovascular disease. Journal of Vascular Surgery. 1988;**8**:721-729

[54] den Hartog AG, Algra A, Moll FL, de Borst GJ. Mechanisms of gender-related outcome differences after carotid endarterectomy. Journal of Vascular Surgery. 2010;**52**:1062-1071.e6. DOI: 10.1016/j.jvs.2010.03.068

[55] Bisdas T, Egorova N, Moskowitz AJ, Sosunov EA, Marin ML, Faries PL, et al. The impact of gender on in-hospital outcomes after carotid endarterectomy or stenting. European Journal of Vascular and Endovascular Surgery. 2012;**44**:244-250. DOI: 10.1016/J.EJVS.2012.06.009

[56] de Waard DD, Halliday A, de Borst GJ, Bulbulia R, Huibers A, Casana R, et al. Choices of stent and cerebral protection in the ongoing ACST-2 trial: A descriptive study. European Journal of Vascular and Endovascular Surgery. 2017;**53**:617-625. DOI: 10.1016/j.ejvs.2016.12.034

[57] Halliday A, Bulbulia R, Gray W, Naughten A, den Hartog A, Delmestri A, Wallis C, le Conte S, Macdonald S. Status update and interim results from the asymptomatic carotid surgery trial-2 (ACST-2). European Journal of Vascular and Endovascular Surgery. 2013; **46**:510-518. DOI: 10.1016/j.ejvs.2013.07.020

[58] Huibers A, Halliday A, Bulbulia R, Coppi G, de Borst GJ. Antiplatelet therapy in carotid artery stenting and carotid endarterectomy in the asymptomatic carotid surgery trial-2. European Journal of Vascular and Endovascular Surgery. 2016;**51**:336-342. DOI: 10.1016/J.EJVS.2015.11.002

Chapter 6

Gender-Associated Biomarkers in Metabolic Syndrome

Rosa Vona, Lucrezia Gambardella and
Elisabetta Straface

Additional information is available at the end of the chapter

http://dx.doi.org/10.5772/intechopen.81103

Abstract

Metabolic syndrome (MetS) is a cluster of risk factors for atherosclerosis, including abdominal obesity, hypertension, insulin resistance, dyslipidemia with high triglycerides, and low high-density lipoprotein cholesterol. Affected patients have a significantly increased risk of developing cardiovascular disorders (CVD), that are the leading cause of death in the Western countries. Several epidemiological studies have investigated the evolution of CVD hypothesizing the presence of a gender difference in the pathogenetic and progression determinants detectable in men and women. In this chapter, we will examine new gender-associated bioindicators of possible diagnostic or prognostic value in the MetS. Moreover, we will provide an overview on current knowledge on sex-associated cardiovascular determinants with the aim to improve CVD diagnostic and prognostic clinical courses and to develop new and gender-biased prevention strategies.

Keywords: metabolic syndrome, biomarkers, gender differences

1. Introduction

This chapter is aimed to detect gender-associated biomarkers in metabolic syndrome (MS), a clustering of several risk factors associated with significant cardiovascular morbidity and mortality. Cardiovascular diseases (CVD) are the first cause of death in the world according to the World Health Organization. Over 17 million people died from CVD in 2015 and the economic burden of CVD each year is estimated at 396 billion dollars in the US, with similar perspective in Europe, and is expected to rise above 1 trillion dollars in 2030 [5]. Several epidemiological studies, the Framingham in particular, have investigated into the evolution of CVD hypothesizing the presence of a gender difference in the pathogenetic and progression determinants detectable in men and women [36]. Metabolic syndrome contributes considerably to cardiovascular mortality, particularly among women [33].

Here, we will examine new gender-associated bioindicators of possible diagnostic or prognostic value in the MS. Moreover, we will provide an overview on current knowledge on sex-associated cardiovascular determinants with the aim to improve CVD diagnostic and prognostic clinical courses and to develop new and gender-biased prevention strategies.

2. Metabolic syndrome

In 1977, Haller used the term "metabolic syndrome" (MS) to describe the association between hypertension, dyslipidemia, obesity, and disturbed glucose metabolism [29]. In particular, he demonstrated how the presence of multiple of these factors increased the risk of developing cardiovascular disease [29]. Some years later, Phillips suggested that the combination of risk factors not only predisposed to heart disease, but was also related with an increased risk for obesity. This cluster of risk factors included glucose intolerance, hyperinsulinemia, and a high level of triglycerides, glucose, cholesterol, and insulin [73]. MS is due to the increase in body mass index (BMI) as result of an increase in caloric intake, increase in obesity percentage, and increased sedentary life habits [96]. As said before, this clinical entity has a cluster of risk factors such as hypertension, central obesity, increased triglycerides, decreased high-density lipoprotein cholesterol (HDL-C), increased blood glucose, and insulin resistance [11, 44]. The prevalence of the MS worldwide is estimated to be between 10 and 84%, highlighting a certain correlation with developed countries, but it also depends on various factors such as socioeconomic status, lifestyle, BMI, and region studied [38, 96]. Moreover, a higher rate was found in urban compared with rural populations [76, 114].

A study by Khosravi-Boroujeni and coworker showed that the prevalence of MS has changed from 2001 to 2013 [41]. They also mentioned that incidence of diabetes has also been increasing over the years. Data from the International Diabetes Federation (IDF) suggested that 25% of worldwide adult population suffer from the syndrome with 5% in those exhibiting normal weight, 22% being overweight, and 60% being obese [52, 114]. This has been attributed to aging, life style changes, population growth, obesity, and decline in physical activity. Central obesity was labeled as a critical component of the MS. The prevalence of the hypertriglyceridemia also declined, due to use of the statins, healthy eating with cutting back on fat [41].

3. Biomarker

3.1. Definition and characteristics

To predict cardiovascular risk, numerous biomarkers have been developed. Some of them are used in medicine to facilitate diagnosis, assess risk, direct therapy, and determine efficacy of treatment. The FDA-NIH Biomarker Working Group in the Biomarkers, Endpoints, and other

Tools (BEST) Resource (https://www.ncbi.nlm.nih.gov/books/NBK326791/) define a biomarker as "a defined characteristic that is measured as an indicator of normal biological processes, pathogenic processes, or responses to an exposure or intervention." A clinically useful biomarker must be able to meet one of the following criteria: (i) show specificity and sensitivity for a certain disease (diagnostic); (ii) have prognostic value; and (iii) correlate with disease activity. Some of them are simple traditional biomarkers based on lipid profile and risk factors [74, 81, 93].

In the INTERHEART study, 9 major risk factors could explain 90% of the population-attributable risk in men and 94% in women of 52 countries. These factors are abdominal obesity, elevated lipids, hypertension, diabetes, smoking, psychosocial factors, consumption of fruits/vegetables, consumption of alcohol, and regular physical activity [110]. However, the importance of these factors varies significantly from one country to another and some of these factors act as predisposing and not causal factors, like obesity and diet [111]. The prevalence of risk factors can change in different directions around the world, often because of socioeconomic and political cues.

Hypertension, central obesity, increased triglycerides, decreased high-density lipoprotein cholesterol (HDL-C), increased blood glucose and insulin resistance are collectively defined as risk factors for cardiovascular disease triggered by metabolic syndrome [11, 44, 62] (**Table 1**). In the last few years, in addition to the clinical factors, new factors in the pathogenesis of MS have also been taken into consideration. These factors can be classified on the basis of their function (e.g., marker of exposition, markers of effects, etc.) or in their biochemical or biologic properties (e.g., proteins metabolites, hormones, cytokines, etc.) [92].

Ample evidence favors a key role for mitochondrial injury, oxidative stress, and apoptosis in MS [7]. Moreover, recent findings depicted an essential role for autophagy, a cellular process of degrading long-lived, injured proteins and organelles, in the pathogenesis of MS [65, 108, 114]. Indeed, dysregulated autophagy is present in multiple metabolic anomalies including obesity, insulin resistance, diabetes mellitus, and dyslipidemia [42, 47, 61, 112, 113].

Recent studies implicated that inflammation, especially chronic low-grade inflammation, might play an even greater role in the development of MS [56]. One possible mechanism is that the growth of adipose tissue and infiltration of immune cells lead to the increase of

Components	International Diabetes Federation
Obesity-waist circumference (cm)	≥35 cm for women or ≥ 40 cm for men
Hypertension-blood pressure (mmHg)	130/85 mm Hg
Dyslipidemia-reduced HDL (mg/dL)	<40 mg/dL in men or < 50 mg/dL in women
Dyslipidemia-elevated triglycerides (mg/dL)	≥150 mg/dL
Glucose-fasting blood glucose (mg/dL)	≥100 mg/dL

HDL: high-density lipoprotein.

Table 1. Current criteria for the diagnosis of the metabolic syndrome.

proinflammatory adipokines such as tumor necrosis factor alpha (TNF-α), C-reactive protein (CRP), and interleukin-6 (IL-6) [37, 59, 104, 105], which cause increased insulin resistance from insulin-sensitive tissues by decreasing insulin signaling [34].

We will present the current state of knowledge for modifiable biomarkers that can be used to predict MS events in the general population.

3.2. Elevated systolic blood pressure

Elevated systolic blood pressure (SBP) is one of the leading risk factors for global mortality and for CVDs. In 2015, the prevalence of raised blood pressure was around 20% in females aged 18 and over 24% in males [100]. Studies have reported conflicting results on the association between increments in SBP and CVDs with differences between sexes [2]. An analysis carried out in 2013 found that every 10 mm Hg increment in SBP was associated with a 15% increased risk of coronary heart disease and a 25% increased risk of stroke in both men and women, indicating a similar impact of hypertension on cardiovascular outcomes in both sexes [71]. In contrast, a recent study on US population indicates that women experienced a 10% greater risk in CVDs per 10 mm Hg increment in SBP than men [103].

3.3. Dyslipidemia

Higher total cholesterol (TC) is estimated to account for over 2.6 million deaths (4.5% of total) worldwide every year [100]. The prevalence of elevated TC is similar in men and women [100] and studies addressing the possible sex-/gender-specific effects of TC on CVD risk have reported inconsistent results [72]. The cholesterol associated with high-density lipoproteins (HDL-C) has long been considered a useful biomarker of CVD and MS risk. In population studies, HDL-C is inversely related to the risk of myocardial infarction and death [57]. Low HDL was initially suggested to be more predictive of coronary risk in women compared to men [82]; however, analyses indicated that the association between HDL cholesterol levels and fatal coronary heart disease did not vary significantly by sex [22]. The first systematic meta-analysis evaluating the impact of TC on CVD risk in women compared with men [72] found that for every 1-mmol/L increment in TC, the risk of coronary heart diseases increased by 20% in women and by 24% in men, indicating essentially a similar TC-related risk of coronary heart diseases in both sexes.

3.4. Triglycerides

Plasma triglycerides (TG) are product in the intestine and in the liver. As elevated TG are often associated with reduced levels of the negative cardiovascular risk biomarker HDL-C, the causal role of elevated plasma TG in CVD has been debated over the last 50 years. Fortunately, different types of genetic and epidemiological evidence have recently strengthened the causality relationship between TG and CVD and promoted TG lowering as a fundamental factor for CVD prevention. The question is important considering the high prevalence of TG levels: 47% of the US population at over 1.7 mmol/L based on the 2011 NHANES survey [10].

Initially, it was thought that TG level was a stronger risk biomarker in women than in men. Some years later, in a meta-analysis of 29 Western prospective studies with 262,525 subjects, a significant association of TG with cardiovascular events was found, which was attenuated by adjusting for HDL-C but remained significant [81, 88].

3.5. Body fat, excess body weight, and obesity

Excess body weight is another major risk factor for CVDs and MS; moreover, excess body weight is currently one of the greatest public health issues worldwide [99]. According to the WHO, over 650 million adults were estimated to be obese worldwide in 2016 and prevalence has almost tripled since 1975 confirming that excess body weight has reached epidemic proportions globally. The association between BMI and coronary heart diseases has been shown to be the same between men and women in several studies [23, 66, 78]. The increased BMI has the same deleterious effects on the risk of MS onset in women and men [11, 62]. However, there are numerous differences between men and women regarding body fat, excess body weight, and obesity that could be due to either direct activation by sex steroids or by sex steroid-independent mechanisms.

3.6. Dysglycemia

Dysglycemia is a global term referring to either impaired fasting glucose or impaired glucose tolerance. However, the two conditions are physiologically distinct. Impaired fasting glucose results from inadequate basal insulin secretion or sensitivity in the liver, whereas impaired glucose tolerance is a consequence of insufficient insulin response or sensitivity to a carbohydrate load in not only the liver but also skeletal muscle. Impaired glucose tolerance is more common in women than in men (except at older ages), whereas impaired fasting glucose is more often seen in men than in women. The reasons for this pattern are unknown, but sex differences in muscle mass, visceral adiposity, altered susceptibility to free fatty acid-induced peripheral insulin resistance, and other factors may play a role [77]. Because impaired glucose tolerance is not included in most current MS definitions, it is possible that, compared with their men counterparts, dysglycemic women are underdiagnosed with the syndrome [77].

3.7. High-sensitivity C-reactive protein

High-sensitivity C-reactive protein (hs-CRP) is a sensitive marker of inflammation. Some findings have indicated that there is an association between CRP, development of atherosclerotic disease [83, 84], and components of the metabolic syndrome [25, 49]. Indeed, many studies have shown a direct association between high concentrations of CRP and insulin resistance or components of MS [17, 27, 39, 53, 87].

While elevated TGs do not exert an inflammatory stimulus per se, endothelial damage may occur, also because of the occurrence of intravascular TGs hydrolysis via the activity of lipoprotein lipase either at the endothelial surface or within the arterial intima. This process leads to a release of free fatty acids and monoacylglycerols which generate local inflammation and high levels of CRP [69, 86].

3.8. Mitochondria functions and its role in MS

Mitochondrial dysfunction is an early pathophysiological event in the development of insulin resistance and obesity [15]. The origin of mitochondrial dysfunction may relate to a variety of processes ranging from inflammation to epigenetic inheritance [48, 94]. Mitochondria are crucial, multifunctional organelles, which actively regulate cellular homeostasis. The main function of mitochondria is the energy production as adenosine triphosphate (ATP) via citric cycle (tricarboxylic acid cycle and Krebs cycle). Other cell functions include ionic homeostasis, production and regulation of reactive oxygen species (ROS), lipid and carbohydrate utilization, pH regulation, steroid hormone synthesis, calcium homeostasis, thermogenesis, and cell death [70, 85, 98]. An intricate homeostatic system regulates and maintains optimal mitochondrial function in healthy cells, the failure of which is seen in obesity, asthma, and metabolic syndrome [6].

Mitochondria are known to adapt physically to nutrient availability [26, 79]. The study's Durigon and coworker demonstrates that changes in nutrient availability and utilization remodel the nucleoprotein complexes in mitochondria and thereby indicates how nutrients can modulate gene expression and energy production in the organelle. It is clear that genetic defects in metabolic factors linked to mitochondrial nucleoprotein complexes, or their regulators, can produce a pseudostarvation state, owing to an inability to utilize an available nutrient [21].

Several cardiovascular risk factors such as type 2 diabetes mellitus, hypertension, atrial fibrillation, peripheral artery disease, obesity, MS, dyslipidemia, habit of smoking, and pollution are associated with an increased production of ROS [75].

The most common cause of obesity, caloric excess, and high fat consumption, leads to nutritional overload, excess electron flux, increased oxidative stress, accumulation of partially oxidized substrates, and, eventually, damage [45, 102]. As mentioned above, mitochondria are the primary intracellular site of oxygen consumption and the major source of reactive oxygen species (ROS), most of them originating from the mitochondrial respiratory chain. These highly reactive molecules, radicals, and nonradicals have the ability to capture electrons from molecules they come in contact with, including proteins and nucleic acids, leading in consequence to cell damage. A fine equilibrium between ROS production and ROS removal determines the physiological versus pathological function of ROS. In fact, an excessive amount of ROS induces oxidative stress and promotes cell death under hypoxic conditions. Conversely, at physiological levels, ROS function as "redox messengers" in intracellular signaling [18, 98]. ROS can be removed by antioxidant enzymes such as superoxide dismutase, catalase, and glutathione peroxidase [18]. An efficient antioxidant system is also necessary to cope with reactive nitric species (RNS) generated by the reaction between O_2^- and nitric oxide (NO) [4]. Similar to ROS, excessive accumulation of RNS leads to irreversible damage to biomolecules [1].

The mitochondrial dysfunction leads to activation of stress pathways that reduce cellular sensitivity to insulin, limiting nutrient influx, and preventing further damage. Chronically, this manifests as reduced mitochondrial metabolism, insulin resistance in organs, such as liver and skeletal muscle, with consequent hyperinsulinemia and diversion of nutrients to storage as adipose tissue [63]. In addition, mitochondrial dysfunction, with rising intracellular oxygen and oxidative stress, interferes with NO synthesis and leads to oxonitrative stress in epithelial and vascular endothelial cells. This pattern underlies the metabolic syndrome with obesity, diabetes, dyslipidemia, and hypertension as the phenotypic components. MS is thought to be related to inflammatory processes and oxidative stress that are linked to underlying adipocyte cellular dysfunction [3, 20].

3.9. Autophagy in MS

Autophagy (or self-eating) is a conserved process aimed at maintaining of cellular and tissue homeostasis under normal as well as stress conditions, including nutrient starvation, changes in metabolism, energy and oxygen status. Autophagy is a degradation mechanism for nonessential or damaged cytoplasmic components, including damaged organelles, toxic protein aggregates, and intracellular pathogens [64]. It is an evolutionarily conserved process, in which cells engulf a portion of the cytoplasm and damaged organelles (such as mitochondria, peroxisomes, and endoplasmic reticulum) into double-membraned vesicles which later fuse with lysosomes for the degradation of enclosed materials [14, 32, 50]. Degradation by-products, such as amino acids, can then be re-used for the building of new macromolecules or for meeting metabolic demands [43, 109]. Autophagy serves as an indispensable process for cellular homeostasis involved in immunity, inflammation, and metabolism [16]. Either excessive or defective autophagy may be associated with human metabolic diseases [91], indicating the unique role of autophagy in the regulation of metabolic homeostasis [114]. Besides the main function of energy production, mitochondria are also able to turn on and tune autophagy by ROS production and oxidation of mitochondrial lipids. Excessive accumulation of ROS leads to impairment of mitochondria structure and function, which in turn triggers a selective process of mitochondria self-removal called mitophagy. As already mentioned, mitophagy is an autophagic response that allows elimination of defective mitochondria and accelerates the mitochondrial turnover, thus preserving the pool of healthy organelles [80]. It has been proposed that upon nutrient deprivation, mitochondria protect themselves from degradation by promoting fusion and inhibiting fission events. It is only after long-term starvation that mitochondria undergo fragmentation and are eventually removed by mitophagy [79]. A reciprocal regulatory mechanism exists between autophagy and key metabolic elements such as glucose and lipids [54, 55, 80]. For example, lipotoxicity in metabolic anomalies impairs lysosomal function and autophagy, further exacerbating lipid accumulation and ultimately cell injury [95]. Autophagy plays a pivotal role in the maintenance of the body's metabolism. Clinical and experimental evidences have depicted a link between autophagy and metabolic risk factors such as obesity, dyslipidemia, alcoholism, insulin resistance, hypertension, diabetes mellitus, sepsis, and inflammation [16, 51, 58, 90, 101, 114]. The bioengineered autophagy models also show a key role of autophagy in systemic metabolic regulation. Specifically, they highlight how not only changes in autophagy affect metabolic homeostasis but also the metabolic stress affects the state of autophagy. Indeed, autophagy is suppressed in genetic or diet-induced models of obesity in various tissues, including liver, skeletal muscle, and cardiac muscle [12, 13, 31, 35, 54, 55, 106, 107]. Recent data show that elevated circulating insulin, an autophagy-inhibitory hormone, is believed to be responsible for changes in autophagy genes [89]. A more in-depth understanding of the role of autophagy in metabolic diseases should yield potential therapeutic strategies for better management of metabolic syndrome.

4. Metabolic syndrome and gender differences

Individuals with MS are four to five times more likely to develop diabetes and about twice as likely to develop CVDs than those without the syndrome [60, 77]. Recently, a meta-analysis of data from five cohorts with a total of 18,353 participants suggested that MS is associated with similar elevations in CVD risk in women and men [77]. It is unclear whether MS confers additional risk beyond its individual components. Comparative data from two U.S. National Health and Nutrition Surveys (NHANES III (1988–1994) and NHANES (1999-2006)) show a striking rise in prevalence of MS, with the relative increase larger in women (22.8%) than in men (11.2%) [68]. In NHANES III, the prevalence of specific risk factor clusters responsible for the MS diagnosis differed between the sexes, at least in the cluster under age 65 [46]. Abdominal obesity was a dominant feature in females with MS, whereas risk factor combinations were more heterogenous in their male counterparts. Sex affects not only the clinical expression but also the pathophysiology of MS. A recent review [77] demonstrates that sex differences in dysglycemia, body fat, adipocyte biology, and the hormonal control of body weight may have a role in cardiometabolic aftermath of women and men with the MS. Moreover, the estrogen decline, that occurs postmenopausally, may have also implications for cardiometabolic sequela in MS women [77].

The sex difference in the distribution of body fat is well known. Specifically, there is an adipose tissue accrual in the upper body (trunk and abdomen) and lower body (hips and thighs) more prominent in men and women, respectively. Visceral adipose tissue in the abdomen is a stronger correlate than subcutaneous adipose tissue of metabolic disturbances and cardiovascular risk. The amount of visceral adipose tissue, as well as the ratio of visceral adipose tissue to total body fat, is lower in premenopausal women than in men. These findings imply that BMI and waist circumference, commonly used in epidemiologic settings, are less accurate indicators of visceral obesity in women and may thus underestimate the impact of visceral adipose tissue on cardiometabolic risk in this group [60].

Sex influences adipocyte size in certain anatomic locations. For example, in men, omental adipocytes (a type of intraperitoneal visceral adipose tissue) and abdominal subcutaneous adipocytes are approximately equal in diameter, and show only minimal size increases with increasing BMI. In contrast, in women, omental adipocytes are 20–30% smaller than abdominal subcutaneous adipocytes, and show larger size increases as BMI increases. Thus, sex differences in adipocyte size may affect the cardiometabolic risk associated with MS in women and men [60].

Sex differences in hormonal control of body weight may also contribute to the clinical expression and sequelae of MS. The hormones insulin, leptin, and estrogen may interact to play a role in weight control via "adiposity signals" to the brain. In particular, insulin is secreted from pancreatic beta cells in response to rising glucose levels. Leptin, which has the effect of inhibiting food intake, suppressing insulin secretion, and increasing lipolysis, is released from adipose tissue in direct proportion to fat mass [19, 30]. Leptin expression is greater in subcutaneous than in visceral adipocytes, whereas insulin is a better marker of visceral than subcutaneous fat [19]. Given the aforementioned sex differences in visceral vs. subcutaneous fat, it seems likely that hormonal control of body weight varies in women and men. Sex differences in adipose tissue are not limited to white adipose depots, as females have more brown adipose tissue and an enhanced capacity to beige their adipose tissue [24].

The mass changes that occur in adipose tissue gene expression in response to diet-induced obesity are different between males and females, demonstrating significant differences in how obesity affects adipose tissue [28].

The estrogen family and its two respective receptors, ERα and ERβ, have been widely suggested to be protective against obesity, type 2 diabetes, and cardiovascular disease [67]. Accumulating data also suggest that estrogen affects adipocyte biology, as well as glucose and lipid metabolism. Estrogens have significant effects on insulin and leptin sensitivity and on the body's response to changes in glucose levels [19, 67]. At menopause, a time of fluctuating and ultimately falling estrogen levels, an increase in visceral adiposity occurs, along with atherogenic lipid changes characteristic of MS [60].

Estrogens can exert significant effects on one important cellular component as mitochondria. Differences in mitochondrial number and function have been suggested to underlie the differences in life span between the sexes [97] and may also be responsible for some of the differences in response to the early life nutritional environment. Females have increased mitochondrial number in skeletal muscle, adipose tissue, and heart [8, 9, 40].

5. Conclusions

Progressive obesity, insulin resistance, abnormal cholesterol, or triglyceride levels that lead to metabolic syndrome are emerging problems. Many strategies have been recently proposed to minimize health-related consequences of metabolic syndrome. Sex seems to be the one element that plays a key role not only in the clinical expression but also in the pathophysiology of MS. The endogenous causes of the sex differences observed in many diseases are largely unknown, and the situation in CVD research is not much different. Much remains to be learned about mechanisms for these sex differences. Gaining this knowledge would allow us to therapeutically target the relevant protective pathways. Sex differences in the clinical expression and physiology of metabolic syndrome may be important in refining predictions of cardiovascular risk.

Author details

Rosa Vona, Lucrezia Gambardella and Elisabetta Straface*

*Address all correspondence to: elisabetta.straface@iss.it

Center for Gender-Specific Medicine, Istituto Superiore di Sanità, Rome, Italy

References

[1] Allen CL, Bayraktutan U. Oxidative stress and its role in the pathogenesis of ischaemic stroke. International Journal of Stroke. 2009;**4**(6):461-470

[2] Appelman Y, van Rijn BB, Ten Haaf ME, Boersma E, Peters SA. Sex differences in cardiovascular risk factors and disease prevention. Atherosclerosis. 2015;**241**(1):211-218

[3] Aroor AR, McKarns S, Demarco VG, Jia G, Sowers JR. Maladaptive immune and inflammatory pathways lead to cardiovascular insulin resistance. Metabolism. 2013;**62**(11): 1543-1552

[4] Beckman JS, Koppenol WH. Nitric oxide, superoxide, and peroxynitrite: The good, the bad, and ugly. The American Journal of Physiology. 1996;**271**(5 Pt 1):C1424-C1437

[5] Benjamin EJ, Blaha MJ, Chiuve SE, Cushman M, Das SR, Deo R, et al. Heart disease and stroke statistics-2017 update: A report from the American Heart Association. Circulation. 2017;**135**(10):e146-e603

[6] Bhatraju NK, Agrawal A. Mitochondrial dysfunction linking obesity and asthma. Annals of the American Thoracic Society. 2017;**14**(Supplement_5):S368-S373

[7] Bhatti JS, Bhatti GK, Reddy PH. Mitochondrial dysfunction and oxidative stress in metabolic disorders—A step towards mitochondria based therapeutic strategies. Biochimica et Biophysica Acta. 2017;**1863**(5):1066-1077

[8] Capllonch-Amer G, Lladó I, Proenza AM, García-Palmer FJ, Gianotti M. Opposite effects of 17-β estradiol and testosterone on mitochondrial biogenesis and adiponectin synthesis in white adipocytes. Journal of Molecular Endocrinology. 2014;**52**(2):203-214

[9] Capllonch-Amer G, Sbert-Roig M, Galmés-Pascual BM, Proenza AM, Lladó I, Gianotti M, et al. Estradiol stimulates mitochondrial biogenesis and adiponectin expression in skeletal muscle. The Journal of Endocrinology. 2014;**221**(3):391-403

[10] Carroll MD, Kit BK, Lacher DA, Shero ST, Mussolino ME. Trends in lipids and lipoproteins in US adults, 1988-2010. JAMA. 2012;**308**(15):1545-1554. DOI: 10.1001/jama.2012.13260

[11] Castaneda A, Jauregui-Maldonado E, Ratnani I, Varon J, Surani S. Correlation between metabolic syndrome and sleep apnea. World Journal of Diabetes. 2018;**9**(4):66-71

[12] Chang E, Kim L, Choi JM, Park SE, Rhee EJ, Lee WY, et al. Ezetimibe stimulates intestinal glucagon-like peptide 1 secretion via the MEK/ERK pathway rather than dipeptidyl peptidase 4 inhibition. Metabolism. 2016;**64**(5):633-641

[13] Chang HH, Moro A, Takakura K, Su HY, Mo A, Nakanishi M, et al. Incidence of pancreatic cancer is dramatically increased by a high fat, high calorie diet in KrasG12D mice. PLoS One. 2017;**12**(9):e0184455

[14] Chen Y, Klionsky DJ. The regulation of autophagy—Unanswered questions. Journal of Cell Science. 2011;**124**(Pt 2):161-170

[15] Cheng Z, Almeida FA. Mitochondrial alteration in type 2 diabetes and obesity: An epigenetic link. Cell Cycle. 2014;**13**(6):890-897

[16] Choi AM, Ryter SW, Levine B. Autophagy in human health and disease. The New England Journal of Medicine. 2013;**368**(19):1845-1846

[17] Choi KM, Ryu OH, Lee KW, Kim HY, Seo JA, Kim SG, et al. Serum adiponectin, interleukin-10 levels and inflammatory markers in the metabolic syndrome. Diabetes Research and Clinical Practice. 2007;**75**(2):235-240

[18] Circu ML, Aw TY. Reactive oxygen species, cellular redox systems, and apoptosis. Free Radical Biology & Medicine. 2010;**48**:749-762

[19] Dearden L, Bouret SG, Ozanne SE. Sex and gender differences in developmental programming of metabolism. Molecular Metabolism. 2018;**15**:8-19

[20] DeBoer MD. Obesity, systemic inflammation, and increased risk for cardiovascular disease and diabetes among adolescents: A need for screening tools to target interventions. Nutrition. 2013;**29**(2):379-386

[21] Durigon R, Mitchell AL, Jones AW, Manole A, Mennuni M, Hirst EM, et al. LETM1 couples mitochondrial DNA metabolism and nutrient preference. EMBO Molecular Medicine. 2018;**10**(9). pii:e8550

[22] Di Angelantonio E, Sarwar N, Perry P, Kaptoge S, Ray KK, Thompson A, et al. Major lipids, apolipoproteins, and risk of vascular disease. JAMA. 2009;**302**(18):1993-2000

[23] Wormser D, Kaptoge S, Di Angelantonio E, Wood AM, Pennells L, Emerging Risk Factors Collaboration. Separate and combined associations of body-mass index and abdominal adiposity with cardiovascular disease: Collaborative analysis of 58 prospective studies. Lancet. 2011;**377**(9771):1085-1095

[24] Frank AP, Palmer BF, Clegg DJ. Do estrogens enhance activation of brown and beiging of adipose tissues? Physiology & Behavior. 2018;**187**:24-31

[25] Fröhlich M, Imhof A, Berg G, Hutchinson WL, Pepys MB, Boeing H, et al. Association between C-reactive protein and features of the metabolic syndrome: A population-based study. Diabetes Care. 2000;**23**(12):1835-1839

[26] Gomes LC, Di Benedetto G, Scorrano L. During autophagy mitochondria elongate, are spared from degradation and sustain cell viability. Nature Cell Biology. 2011;**13**(5):589-598

[27] González AS, Guerrero DB, Soto MB, Díaz SP, Martinez-Olmos M, Vidal O. Metabolic syndrome, insulin resistance and the inflammation markers C-reactive protein and ferritin. European Journal of Clinical Nutrition. 2006;**60**(6):802-809

[28] Grove KL, Fried SK, Greenberg AS, Xiao XQ, Clegg DJ. A microarray analysis of sexual dimorphism of adipose tissues in high-fat diet-induced obese mice. International Journal of Obesity (London). 2010;**34**:989e1000

[29] Haller H. Epidermiology and associated risk factors of hyperlipoproteinemia. Zeitschrift fur die Gesamte Innere Medizin und Ihre Grenzgebiete. 1977;**32**:124-128

[30] Havel PJ, Kasim-Karakas S, Dubuc GR, Mueller W, Phinney SD. Gender differences in plasma leptin concentrations. Nature Medicine. 1996;**2**:949e950

[31] He C, Bassik MC, Moresi V, Sun K, Wei Y, Zou Z, et al. Exercise-induced BCL2-regulated autophagy is required for muscle glucose homeostasis. Nature. 2012;**481**(7382):511-515

[32] He C, Klionsky DJ. Regulation mechanisms and signaling pathways of autophagy. Annual Review of Genetics. 2009;**43**:67-93

[33] Hess PL, Al-Khalidi HR, Friedman DJ, Mulder H, Kucharska-Newton A, Rosamond WR, et al. The metabolic syndrome and risk of sudden cardiac death: The atherosclerosis risk in communities study. Journal of the American Heart Association. 2017;**6**(8):pii: e006103

[34] Hotamisligil GS, Peraldi P, Budavari A, Ellis R, White MF, Spiegelman BM. IRS-1-mediated inhibition of insulin receptor tyrosine kinase activity in TNF-alpha- and obesity-induced insulin resistance. Science. 1996;**271**(5249):665-668

[35] Hsu HC, Liu CH, Tsai YC, Li SJ, Chen CY, Chu CH, et al. Time dependent cellular response in the liver and heart in a dietary-induced obese mouse model: The potential role of ER stress and autophagy. European Journal of Nutrition. 2016;**55**:2031-2043

[36] Ingelsson E, Pencina MJ, Tofler GH, Benjamin EJ, Lanier KJ, Jacques PF, et al. Multimarker approach to evaluate the incidence of the metabolic syndrome and longitudinal changes in metabolic risk factors: The Framingham offspring study. Circulation. 2007;**116**(9):984-992

[37] Jo J, Gavrilova O, Pack S, Jou W, Mullen S, Sumner AE, et al. Hypertrophy and/or hyperplasia: Dynamics of adipose tissue growth. PLoS Computational Biology. 2009;**5**(3):e1000324

[38] Kaur J. A comprehensive review on metabolic syndrome. Cardiology Research and Practice. 2014;**2014**:943162

[39] Kerner A, Avizohar O, Sella R, Bartha P, Zinder O, Markiewicz W, et al. Association between elevated liver enzymes and C-reactive protein: Possible hepatic contribution to systemic inflammation in the metabolic syndrome. Arteriosclerosis, Thrombosis, and Vascular Biology. 2005;**25**(1):193-197

[40] Khalifa AR, Abdel-Rahman EA, Mahmoud AM, Ali MH, Noureldin M, Saber SH, et al. Sex-specific differences in mitochondria biogenesis, morphology, respiratory function, and ROS homeostasis in young mouse heart and brain. Physiological Reports. 2017;**5**(6):pii: e13125

[41] Khosravi-Boroujeni H, Sarrafzadegan N, Sadeghi M, Roohafza H, Talaei M, Ng SK, et al. Secular trend of metabolic syndrome and its components in a cohort of Iranian adults from 2001 to 2013. Metabolic Syndrome and Related Disorders. 2017;**15**:137-144

[42] Kim KH, Lee MS. Autophagy—A key player in cellular and body metabolism. Nature Reviews. Endocrinology. 2014;**10**(6):322-337

[43] Koleini N, Kardami E. Autophagy and mitophagy in the context of doxorubicin-induced cardiotoxicity. Oncotarget. 2017;**8**(28):46663-46680

[44] Kostoglou-Athanassiou I, Athanassiou P. Metabolic syndrome and sleep apnea. Hippokratia. 2008;**12**:81-86

[45] Koves TR, Ussher JR, Noland RC, Slentz D, Mosedale M, Ilkayeva O, et al. Mitochondrial overload and incomplete fatty acid oxidation contribute to skeletal muscle insulin resistance. Cell Metabolism. 2008;**7**(1):45-56

[46] Kuk JL, Ardern CI. Age and sex differences in the clustering of metabolic syndrome factors: Association with mortality risk. Diabetes Care. 2010;**33**:2457-2461

[47] Lamb CA, Dooley HC, Tooze SA. Endocytosis and autophagy: Shared machinery for degradation. BioEssays. 2013;**35**(1):34-45

[48] Lee HK, Park KS, Cho YM, Lee YY, Pak YK. Mitochondria-based model for fetal origin of adult disease and insulin resistance. Annals of the New York Academy of Sciences. 2005;**1042**:1-18

[49] Lemieux I, Pascot A, Prud'homme D, Alméras N, Bogaty P, Nadeau A, et al. Elevated C-reactive protein: Another component of the atherothrombotic profile of abdominal obesity. Arteriosclerosis, Thrombosis, and Vascular Biology. 2001;**21**(6):961-967

[50] Levine B, Kroemer G. Autophagy in aging, disease and death: The true identity of a cell death impostor. Cell Death and Differentiation. 2012;**16**:1-2

[51] Levine B, Packer M, Codogno P. Development of autophagy inducers in clinical medicine. The Journal of Clinical Investigation. 2015;**125**(1):14-24

[52] Li J, Pfeffer SR. Lysosomal membrane glycoproteins bind cholesterol and contribute to lysosomal cholesterol export. eLife. 2016;**5**:e21635

[53] Lim S, Lee HK, Kimm KC, Park C, Shin C, Cho NH. C-reactive protein level as an independent risk factor of metabolic syndrome in the Korean population. CRP as risk factor of metabolic syndrome. Diabetes Research and Clinical Practice. 2005;**70**(2):126-133

[54] Liu H, Javaheri A, Godar RJ, Murphy J, Ma X, Rohatgi N, et al. Intermittent fasting preserves beta-cell mass in obesity-induced diabetes via the autophagy-lysosome pathway. Autophagy. 2017;**13**(11):1952-1968

[55] Liu L, Liao JZ, He XX, Li PY. The role of autophagy in hepatocellular carcinoma: Friend or foe. Oncotarget. 2017;**8**(34):57707-57722

[56] Lopez-Candales A, Hernández Burgos PM, Hernandez-Suarez DF, Harris D. Linking chronic inflammation with cardiovascular disease: From normal aging to the metabolic syndrome. Journal of Natural Sciences. 2017;**3**(4):pii: e341

[57] Lüscher TF, Landmesser U, von Eckardstein A, Fogelman AM. High-density lipoprotein: Vascular protective effects, dysfunction, and potential as therapeutic target. Circulation Research. 2014;**114**(1):171-182

[58] Ma H, Guo R, Yu L, Zhang Y, Ren J. Aldehyde dehydrogenase 2 (ALDH2) rescues myocardial ischaemia/reperfusion injury: Role of autophagy paradox and toxic aldehyde. European Heart Journal. 2011;**32**(8):1025-1038

[59] Ma K, Jin X, Liang X, Zhao Q, Zhang X. Inflammatory mediators involved in the progression of the metabolic syndrome. Diabetes/Metabolism Research and Reviews. 2012;**28**(5):388-394

[60] Manson JE, Bassuk SS. Biomarkers of cardiovascular disease risk in women. Metabolism. 2015;**64**(3 Suppl 1):S33-S39

[61] Marasco MR, Linnemann AK. β-cell autophagy in diabetes pathogenesis. Endocrinology. 2018;**159**(5):2127-2141

[62] Marjani A. A review on metabolic syndrome. Journal of Endocrinology and Metabolism. 2012;**2**(4-5):166-170

[63] Martin SD, McGee SL. The role of mitochondria in the aetiology of insulin resistance and type 2 diabetes. Biochimica et Biophysica Acta. 2014;**1840**(4):1303-1312

[64] Mizushima N, Levine B, Cuervo AM, Klionsky DJ. Autophagy fights disease through cellular self-digestion. Nature. 2008;**451**:1069-1075

[65] Mizushima N. A brief history of autophagy from cell biology to physiology and disease. Nature Cell Biology. 2018;**20**(5):521-527

[66] Mongraw-Chaffin ML, Peters SAE, Huxley RR, Woodward M. The sex-specific association between BMI and coronary heart disease: A systematic review and meta-analysis of 95 cohorts with 1.2 million participants. The Lancet Diabetes and Endocrinology. 2015;**3**(6):437-449

[67] Morselli E, Santos RS, Criollo A, Nelson MD, Palmer BF, Clegg DJ. The effects of estrogens and their receptors on cardiometabolic health. Nature Reviews Endocrinology. 2017;**13**:352e364

[68] Mozumdar A, Liguori G. Persistent increase of prevalence of metabolic syndrome among U.S. adults: NHANES III to NHANES 1999-2006. Diabetes Care. 2011;**34**:216-219

[69] Nordestgaard BG. Triglyceride-rich lipoproteins and atherosclerotic cardiovascular disease: New insights from epidemiology, genetics, and biology. Circulation Research. 2016;**118**(4):547-563

[70] Palmeira CM, Moreno AJ. Mitochondrial Bioenergetics. Methods and Protocols, Methods in Molecular Biology. Vol. 810. New York, NY, USA: Springer; 2012. ISBN:978-1-61779-381-3

[71] Peters SA, Huxley RR, Woodward M. Comparison of the sex-specific associations between systolic blood pressure and the risk of cardiovascular disease: A systematic review and meta-analysis of 124 cohort studies, including 1.2 million individuals. Stroke. 2013;**44**(9):2394-2401

[72] Peters SA, Singhateh Y, Mackay D, Huxley RR, Woodward M. Total cholesterol as a risk factor for coronary heart disease and stroke in women compared with men: A systematic review and meta-analysis. Atherosclerosis. 2016;**248**:123-131

[73] Phillips GB. Sex hormones, risk factors and cardiovascular disease. The American Journal of Medicine. 1978;**65**:7-11

[74] Pietraforte D, Straface E, Piscopo P, Vona R, Confaloni A. Sex-related biomarkers in cardiovascular and neurodegenerative disorders. Annali dell'Istituto Superiore di Sanità. 2016;**52**(2):230-239

[75] Pignatelli P, Menichelli D, Pastori D, Violi F. Oxidative stress and cardiovascular disease: New insights. Kardiologia Polska. 2018;**76**(4):713-722

[76] Pradeepa R, Surendar J, Indulekha K, Chella S, Anjana RM, Mohan V. Prevalence of metabolic syndrome and its association with coronary artery disease among an urban elderly south Indian population (CURES-145). The Journal of the Association of Physicians of India. 2016;**64**:20-25

[77] Pradhan AD. Sex differences in the metabolic syndrome: Implications for cardiovascular health in women. Clinical Chemistry. 2014;**60**:44-52

[78] Whitlock G, Lewington S, Sherliker P, Clarke R, Emberson J, Prospective Studies Collaboration, et al. Body-mass index and cause-specific mortality in 900 000 adults: Collaborative analyses of 57 prospective studies. Lancet. 2009;**373**(9669):1083-1096

[79] Rambold AS, Kostelecky B, Elia N, Lippincott-Schwartz J. Tubular network formation protects mitochondria from autophagosomal degradation during nutrient starvation. Proceedings of the National Academy of Sciences of the United States of America. 2011;**108**(25):10190-10195

[80] Ren J, Taegtmeyer H. Too much or not enough of a good thing—The Janus faces of autophagy in cardiac fuel and protein homeostasis. Journal of Molecular and Cellular Cardiology. 2015;**84**:223-226

[81] Rhainds D, Brodeur MR, Tardif JC. Lipids, apolipoproteins, and inflammatory biomarkers of cardiovascular risk: what have we learned? Clinical Pharmacology and Therapeutics. 2018;**104**(2):244-256

[82] Rich-Edwards JW, Manson JE, Hennekens CH, Buring JE. The primary prevention of coronary heart disease in women. The New England Journal of Medicine. 1995; **332**(26):1758-1766

[83] Ridker PM, Hennekens CH, Buring JE, Rifai N. C-reactive protein and other markers of inflammation in the prediction of cardiovascular disease in women. The New England Journal of Medicine. 2000;**342**(12):836-843

[84] Ridker PM. High-sensitivity C-reactive protein: Potential adjunct for global risk assessment in the primary prevention of cardiovascular disease. Circulation. 2001;**103**(13): 1813-1818

[85] Rossier MF. T channels and steroid biosynthesis: In search of a link with mitochondria. Cell Calcium. 2006;**40**:155-164

[86] Ruscica M, Ferri N, Macchi C, Corsini A, Sirtori CR. Lipid lowering drugs and inflammatory changes: An impact on cardiovascular outcomes? Annals of Medicine. 2018;**6**:1-46

[87] Sarbijani HM, Marjani A, Khoshnia M. The association between metabolic syndrome and serum levels of adiponectin and high sensitive C reactive protein in Gorgan. Endocrine, Metabolic & Immune Disorders Drug Targets. 2016;**16**(2):107-112

[88] Sarwar N, Danesh J, Eiriksdottir G, Sigurdsson G, Wareham N, Bingham S, et al. Triglycerides and the risk of coronary heart disease: 10,158 incident cases among 262,525 participants in 29 Western prospective studies. Circulation. 2007;**115**(4):450-458

[89] Settembre C, De Cegli R, Mansueto G, Saha PK, Vetrini F, Visvikis O, et al. TFEB controls cellular lipid metabolism through a starvation-induced autoregulatory loop. Nature Cell Biology. 2013;**15**(6):647-658

[90] Sinha RA, Singh BK, Yen PM. Reciprocal crosstalk between autophagic and endocrine signaling in metabolic homeostasis. Endocrine Reviews. 2017;**38**(1):69-102

[91] Sinha-Hikim AP, Sinha-Hikim I, Friedman TC. Connection of nicotine to diet-induced obesity and non-alcoholic fatty liver disease: Cellular and mechanistic insights. Frontiers in Endocrinology. 2017;**8**:23

[92] Straface E, Gambardella L, Canali E, Metere A, Gabrielli N, Arcieri R, et al. P-selectin as a new gender associated biomarker in patients with metabolic syndrome. International Journal of Cardiology. 2010;**145**(3):570-571

[93] Straface E, Malorni W, Pietraforte D. Sex differences in redox biology: A mandatory new point of view approaching human inflammatory diseases. Antioxidants & Redox Signaling. 2017;**26**(1):44-45

[94] Szendroedi J, Phielix E, Roden M. The role of mitochondria in insulin resistance and type 2 diabetes mellitus. Nature Reviews. Endocrinology. 2011;**8**(2):92-103

[95] Taniguchi H, Tanisawa K, Sun X, Kubo T, Higuchi M. Endurance exercise reduces hepatic fat content and serum fibroblast growth factor 21 levels in elderly men. The Journal of Clinical Endocrinology and Metabolism. 2016;**101**(1):191-198

[96] Thounaojam MC, Nammi S, Jadeja R. Natural products for the treatment of obesity, metabolic syndrome, and type 2 diabetes 2016. Evidence-based Complementary and Alternative Medicine. 2016;**2016**:9072345

[97] Tower J. Sex-specific regulation of aging and apoptosis. Mechanisms of Ageing and Development. 2006;**127**:705e718

[98] Vona R, Ascione B, Malorni W, Straface E. Mitochondria and sex-specific cardiac function. Advances in Experimental Medicine and Biology. 2018;**1065**:241-256

[99] W.H.O. Cardiovascular Diseases, Fact Sheet. 2017. http://www.who.int/mediacentre/factsheets/fs317/en/

[100] W.H.O. Raised Blood Pressure. Situation and Trends. 2015. http://www.who.int/gho/ncd/risk_factors/blood_pressure_text/en/

[101] Wang S, Ren J. Role of autophagy and regulatory mechanisms in alcoholic cardiomyopathy. Biochimica et Biophysica Acta. 2018;**1864**(6 Pt A):2003-2009

[102] Watt MJ, Hevener AL. Fluxing the mitochondria to insulin resistance. Cell Metabolism. 2008;**7**(1):5-6

[103] Wei YC, George NI, Chang CW, Hicks KA. Assessing sex differences in the risk of cardiovascular disease and mortality per increment in systolic blood pressure: A systematic review and meta-analysis of follow-up studies in the United States. PLoS One. 2017;**12**(1):e0170218

[104] Weisberg SP, McCann D, Desai M, Rosenbaum M, Leibel RL, Ferrante AW Jr. Obesity is associated with macrophage accumulation in adipose tissue. The Journal of Clinical Investigation. 2003;**112**(12):1796-1808

[105] Xu H, Barnes GT, Yang Q, Tan G, Yang D, Chou CJ, et al. Chronic inflammation in fat plays a crucial role in the development of obesity-related insulin resistance. The Journal of Clinical Investigation. 2003;**112**(12):1821-1830

[106] Xu X, Hua Y, Nair S, Zhang Y, Ren J. Akt2 knockout preserves cardiac function in high-fat diet-induced obesity by rescuing cardiac autophagosome maturation. Journal of Molecular Cell Biology. 2013;**5**:61-63

[107] Xu X, Ren J. Macrophage migration inhibitory factor (MIF) knockout preserves cardiac homeostasis through alleviating Akt-mediated myocardial autophagy suppression in high-fat diet-induced obesity. International Journal of Obesity. 2015;**39**:387-396

[108] Yan S, Huda N, Khambu B, Yin XM. Relevance of autophagy to fatty liver diseases and potential therapeutic applications. Amino Acids. 2017;**49**(12):1965-1979

[109] Yin Z, Pascual C, Klionsky DJ. Autophagy: Machinery and regulation. Microbial Cell. 2016;**3**:588-596

[110] Yusuf S, Hawken S, Ounpuu S, Dans T, Avezum A, Lanas F, et al. Effect of potentially modifiable risk factors associated with myocardial infarction in 52 countries (the INTERHEART study): Case-control study. Lancet. 2004;**364**(9438):937-952

[111] Yusuf S, Reddy S, Ounpuu S, Anand S. Global burden of cardiovascular diseases: Part II: Variations in cardiovascular disease by specific ethnic groups and geographic regions and prevention strategies. Circulation. 2001;**104**(23):2855-2864

[112] Zhang Y, Sowers JR, Ren J. Targeting autophagy in obesity: From pathophysiology to management. Nature Reviews. Endocrinology. 2018;**14**(6):356-376

[113] Zhang Y, Whaley-Connell AT, Sowers JR, Ren J. Autophagy as an emerging target in cardiorenal metabolic disease: From pathophysiology to management. Pharmacology & Therapeutics. 2018;**S0163-7258**(18):30106-30102

[114] Zhang Y, Ye P, Luo L, Bai Y, Xu R, Xiao W, et al. Association between arterial stiffness and risk of coronary artery disease in a community-based population. Chinese Medical Journal. 2014;**127**(22):3944-3947

Chapter 7

Carotid Intern Aneurysms

Eduardo Waihrich, Bruno Parente, Paulo Gonçalves,
Fabio Fernandes, Carlos Ontiveros,
Camila Ribeiro and Elias Rabahi

Additional information is available at the end of the chapter

http://dx.doi.org/10.5772/intechopen.81400

Abstract

Cerebral aneurysms (CA) are acquired lesions, affecting 5–10% of the population, being about three times more common in women than in men. The absolute majority of CA is asymptomatic. However, in symptomatic cases, cerebral aneurysms present without about 80% of cases with severe intracranial hemorrhage, with mortality up to 50% and severe morbidity of up to 80%. At this point, the carotid siphon is particularly important because it is the blood gateway to the anterior cerebral circulation, being the most sinuous portion of the internal carotid artery, and because it houses about 30% of the intracranial aneurysm. The constant interactions of blood flow with carotid siphon curvatures are apparently intrinsically related to the epidemiology of these lesions in the various locations of the intracranial circulation and their presentation form. It is well established that a greater anterior knee angle has a significant independent relation with intracranial aneurysms located after carotid siphon, larger aneurysms, and greater risk of rupture. These findings may be associated with the hemodynamic interactions of blood flow and the curvature of carotid siphon. Little is known about the anatomical changes in carotid siphon and, consequently, the repercussions of the hemodynamic changes that the neurosurgical interventions mechanisms could entail. Devices such as intracranial stents, detachable coils, and even clips of aneurysms can modify the morphology of carotid siphon, and the knowledge of these consequences could be used to obtain better therapeutic results. In the last 10 years, a new device for the treatment of intracranial aneurysms has been presenting promising results, flow diverters stents (FDS), and its use to treat aneurysms in carotid siphon appears to cause morphological changes characterized by increased anterior and posterior angles. Specifically, the anterior angle increase was associated with better angiographic results. Aneurysms of the extracranial carotid artery (ECAA) are rare and little is known about its natural history. The etiology is diverse and most ECAA are asymptomatic, but they may progress to a pulsatile mass, cranial nerve compression, or cause a stroke. ECAA treatment is still controversial and a better insight into natural history and risk of complications of the different treatments is needed in order to get the consensus.

Keywords: carotid intern aneurysms, carotid siphon, flow redirecting stents

1. Introduction

1.1. Epidemiological aspects

Cerebral aneurysms (CA) are acquired lesions, characterized as saccular or diffuse dilation of the intracranial arteries walls. It affects 5–10% of the population, being about three times more often in women than in men [1]. About 70–75% of the patients present single lesions and the remains show multiple lesions, which can affect both hemispheres in both the carotid as well as the vertebro-basilar circulation [2].

The absolute majority of CA is asymptomatic. Among the symptomatic patients, about 80% present as hemorrhagic stroke and are characterized by spontaneous subarachnoid hemorrhages. The remaining 20% may present symptoms such as mass effect, thromboembolic events, or nonspecific headaches [3].

Spontaneous subarachnoid hemorrhage (SAH) secondary to CA rupture is commonly described as a devastating disease, accounting for about 5% of all strokes, with an incidence of 10 cases per 100,000 individuals. Vlak et al. showed that the prevalence of unruptured intracranial aneurysms was significantly higher in patients aged 30 years or older compared with those who were younger than 30 years [47]. Autopsy reports have demonstrated that the incidence of SAH or unruptured intracranial aneurysms was 3–4 times higher in patients older than 70 years and that the prevalence of aneurysms increases with aging, as well as prolonged exposure to hypertension, smoking, and atherosclerotic vessel degeneration [48]. The incidence peak is between 50 and 60 years (only 20% of cases occur before 45 years) and there is considerable predominance for females: 1.6 females for 1 male. This female predominance is probably due to hormonal changes, particularly estrogen considering primiparous views or patients with later menarche that present a risk reduction [4, 5]. Epidemiological studies show that the female preponderance of intracranial aneurysms becomes significant only after the fourth or fifth decade, during the perimenopausal and postmenopausal periods. Moreover, estrogen has a protective effect against vascular injury [46] and hormone-replacement therapy has been shown to be a protective factor for subarachnoid hemorrhage [47].

1.2. Risk factors

The exact etiology of CA formation remains unclear. However, there is no doubt that CA are acquired lesions, initiated from a lesion with genetic, atherosclerotic, traumatic, or inflammatory origin in the vascular endothelium and developed by hemodynamic stress in this region [6]. Factors such as blood hypertension, use of oral contraceptives, drugs (cigarette, cocaine, and alcohol), pregnancy, and neurosurgical diagnostic procedures (lumbar puncture and cerebral angiography) are classically associated with the development of lesions or aneurysmal rupture [6–8]. In addition, environmental and geographic factors, such as season and colder territories, increase the incidence of rupture [6–8]. Some genetic syndromes are associated with a higher incidence, such as autosomal dominant polycystic kidney disease type I and II, Marfan syndrome, neurofibromatosis type I, and Ehlers-Danlos syndrome type

II and IV [8]. Patients who have already been treated for a ruptured aneurysm also have an increased risk of developing another lesion, around 2% per year, against 1% of the general population [6–9]. Genetic inheritance related to aneurysmal development has been complex and multigenic; genes such as 1p34.4-36.13, 7q11, 19q13.3, Xp22, endothelial nitric oxide synthase gene, among others, have been frequently found in familial cases of CA [9].

It is believed that these factors converge to modify the intimal layer and increase the hemodynamic stress of the arterial wall. Hemodynamic stress is basically executed by the elements of blood flow and water hammer pulse, which explains the preferential location of the saccular aneurysms in bifurcations and convexities of vascular curvatures, facing the direction that the flow would be if there were no curves [10]. Thus, we can systematize the hemodynamic interaction as the flow inertial force, perpendicular to the arterial wall, and the parallel shear force caused by the viscosity and friction of the blood elements with the arterial wall [10]. The way these forces interact in the formation, development, and rupture of aneurysmal lesions is still a matter of debate, but apparently the shear stress would be more important at the initial moments of aneurysmal formation; whereas, the flow inertial force would be more important for late development and rupture of the lesions [11].

Considering these factors, the carotid siphon deserves special importance, since it is the blood flow gateway to the anterior cerebral circulation, being characteristically the most sinuous portion of the internal carotid artery and with the anterior communicating complex, compound 80% of the CA [4, 10].

1.3. The carotid siphon

The carotid siphon corresponds to the portion of the internal carotid artery that begins at the end of its petrous (horizontal) segment (or lacerum segment) and ends at the supraclinoid internal carotid bifurcation. The first portion, the end of the petrous segment, is characterized by the path of the carotid when exiting its exclusively intraosseous path and traversing the crease of dura mater around the foramen lacerum. This portion may have branches not easily visible angiographically, among which it can be highlighted the coraco-tympanic branch and the artery of the pterygoid canal (vidian artery) [12].

The carotid artery enters the cavernous sinus after crossing the petrolingual ligament, where it presents initially a vertical ascending segment and then we observe the first important curvature, the posterior angle, of about 90° in anterior direction. It is followed by a horizontal intra-cavernous portion, which ends at a second curvature, the anterior angle, with about 160° in upward and posterior direction. In its intracavernosal path, usually arises the meningohypophyseal trunk, close to its first curvature, and then the inferolateral trunk in the extension of its horizontal segment [13].

After the second curvature, the internal carotid crosses two dural rings and emerges to a new horizontal segment, but now supraclinoid and intradural, where it launches its main branches (ophthalmic artery, posterior communicating artery, and anterior choroidal artery), ending with its bifurcation. This bifurcation gives rise to the middle cerebral artery and the anterior cerebral artery, which also marks the end of the carotid siphon [14] (**Figure 1**).

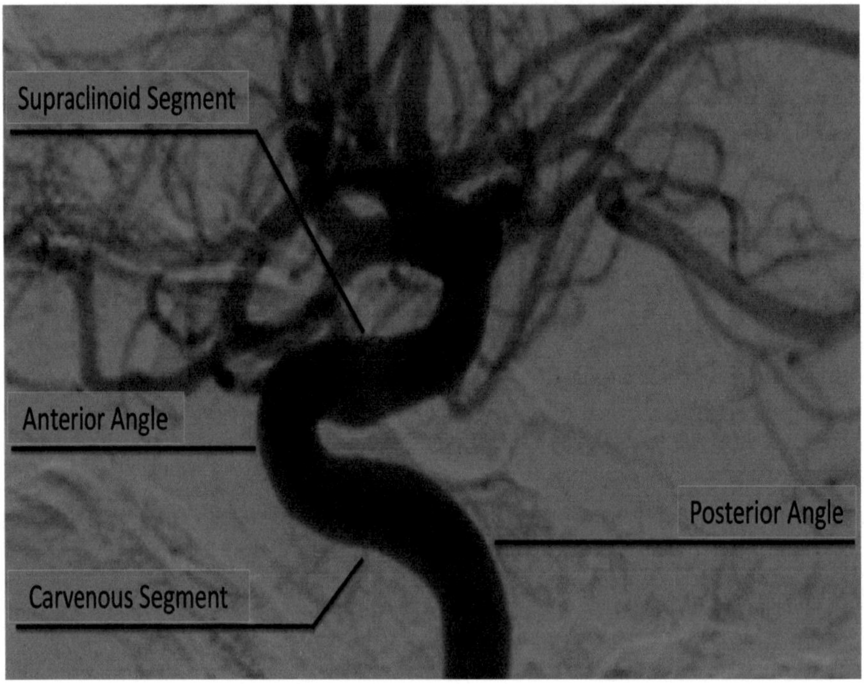

Figure 1. Carotid siphon: digital angiography with subtraction in profile incidence evidencing the segments of the carotid siphon (personal file).

Although this pattern is relativity monotonous among individuals, important anterior and posterior angles variations were identified. These variations were initially systematized by Krayenbuehl and Yasargil, who classified the carotid siphons from the purely morphological point of view into seven subtypes [15] (**Figure 2**):

- Type U, representing 40.1% in the population up to 20 years, 35% between 21 and 50 years, and 15.2% between 51 and 74 years;
- Type V, representing 14.6% in the population up to 20 years, 24.5% between 21 and 50 years, and 22.3% between 51 and 74 years;
- Type C, representing 45.2% in the population up to 20 years, 14.6% between 21 and 50 years, and 5.2% between 51 and 74 years;
- Type Omega, absent up to 20 years, representing 23.7% in the population between 21 and 50 years, and 50.7% between 51 and 74 years;
- Type Double Siphon, absent up to 20 years, representing 1.4% in the population between 21 and 50 years, and 4.1% between 51 and 74 years;
- Type Megasiphon, absent up to 20 years, representing 0.2% in the population between 21 and 50 years, and 2.3% between 51 and 74 years; and
- Type Dolicosiphon, absent up to 20 years, representing 0.4% in the population between 21 and 50 years, and 1.5% between 51 and 74 years.

Subsequently, this classification was reviewed by Zhong, simplifying and systematizing the classification in only four anatomical subtypes of the carotid siphon [16] (**Figure 3**):

- Type U (about 55% of cases): rectified supraclinoid portion with posterior angle greater than 0° and presenting a wide anterior angle of positive values;
- Type V (about 27% of cases): rectified supraclinoid portion with posterior angle greater than 0° and presenting a sharp anterior angle of positive values;
- Type C (about 16% of cases): curved supraclinoid portion, with posterior angle around 0° and presenting a wide anterior angle of negative values; and
- Type S (about 2% of cases): supraclinoid portion rectified with very acute or negative posterior angle, anterior angles of negative values and presenting a wide anterior angle.

The first attempt at geometric and mathematical systematization of the carotid siphon was performed by Lang and Reiter [17], who classified the carotid siphons into three subtypes, exclusively due to the posterior angle. Thus, the most frequent type, 49.3% of the cases, had the posterior angle around 90°. The second subtype, 36.0% of the cases, presented the inferior angle to 90° and the third subtype, 14.7%, with an angle greater than 90°.

This morphology of the siphon is not static and progressively varies with aging, development, and degenerative processes, especially by the influence from atherosclerotic and hypertensive disease [18].

It is believed that the main physiological function of these successive curvatures would be the attenuation of the vectorial force of the blood flow, with consequent reduction of hemodynamic stress to the distal cerebral circulation [18–20]. Thus, there is a constant interaction between the carotid siphon vascular walls with the shear force of the blood elements and the water hammer pulse of the arterial flow [19, 20].

1.4. Wall stressing stress

The consequences that the curvatures of the cerebral circulation generate in the hemodynamics of the carotid siphon, as well as the relation between the incidence of aneurysms and stenoses close to the regions of pronounced curvatures, have been studied in recent years [19, 20].

It is admitted that the loss of the kinetic energy of linear blood flow, when colliding with the endothelial wall of the curvatures, forcing the change of direction of blood flow and transforming the normally linear flow into turbulent flow, is related to the endothelial transformation [18, 21–23]. This phenomenon generates deceleration of the blood flow, reducing the interactions of tangential forces with the vessel wall, called wall shear stress [22].

Recent studies have evidenced the direct relation of the incidence of intracranial stenoses in follow-up with low or oscillatory wall shear stress [23–25]. The characterization of which curvatures and anatomies are more prone to the pathological scenarios has motivated several studies that seek to define the geometric risk factors [24–26]. Piccinelli et al., for example, have shown that curvatures with small radius and low angulation tend to be related to the presence of ruptured aneurysms [27]. Kim and Kang, on the other hand, have demonstrated

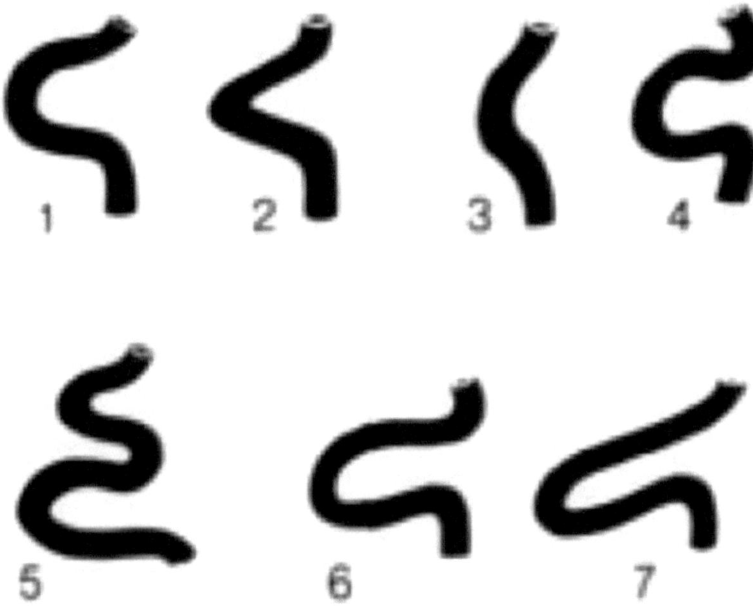

Figure 2. Types of carotid siphon described by Krayenbuehl and Yasargil. (1) Type U, (2) Type V, (3) Type C, (4) Type Omega, (5) Type Double Siphon, (6) Type Megasiphon, and (7) Type Dolicosiphon.

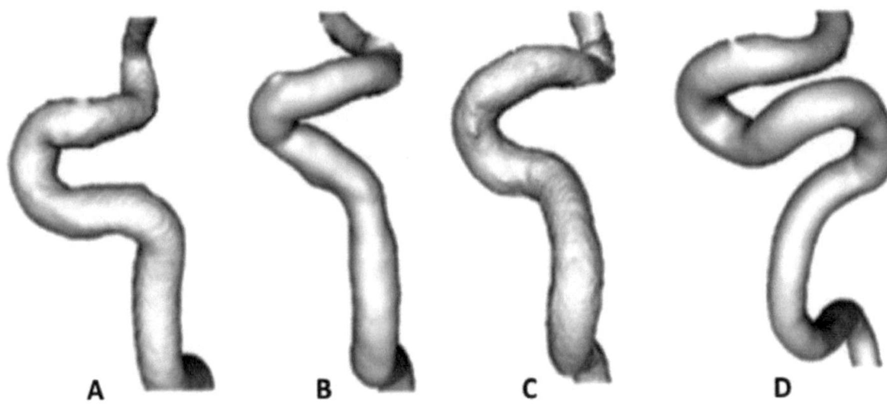

Figure 3. Types of siphons described by Zhong. (A) Type U, (B) Type V, (C) Type C, and (D) Type S [16].

that a short supraclinoid segment of the internal carotid artery is directly associated with an increased incidence of aneurysm of the posterior communicating segment [28]. Zhang et al. have showed that siphons that present more acute curvatures lead to a significant decrease and oscillation of wall shear stress right after curvatures, which are the most favorable sites for the development of stenoses [29]. Silva Neto et al., on the other hand, evidenced that more acute anterior angles are statistically related to a higher incidence of aneurysms in the posterior communicating segment [30]. Sangalli described the association between aneurysms in the most distal portions of the carotid siphon and the less acute curvatures [31]. We recently published our study, where we saw a significant independent direct relation of greater anterior knee angle with intracranial aneurysms located after the carotid siphon, larger aneurysms, and greater risk of rupture. These findings may be associated with the hemodynamic interactions of blood flow and the curvature of the carotid siphon [49].

Anterior angles above the median of our sample (15.40°) are directly related independently to a 36% higher incidence of rupture (p = 0.0055, PR = 1.36, 95% CI: 1.09 to the location of cerebral aneurysms 48% more frequently after the carotid siphon (p = 0.0336, RC = 1.48, 95% CI: 1.03–2.13), and to larger lesions. For each increase of 1° in the anterior angle, there is an increase in aneurysm size of 1001 mm (p = 0.015). These findings may mean that carotid siphons with more intense curvatures would lead to greater changes in the shear force of the wall and greater damping of the vector force in a hammer water pulse. These changes in blood flow would lead to increased hemodynamic stress in the carotid siphon, with a consequent higher frequency of aneurysm in this topography and the formation of smaller lesions and with a lower risk of rupture, due to the decrease in the vector force in a hammer water pulse toward the aneurysmal domus [49].

Then, the change of direction of blood flow at the points of curvature of the carotid siphon occur in detriment of the deceleration of the linear velocity of blood flow and the loss of the linear vector force of the water hammer pulse. This deceleration would occur with a change from laminar to turbulent flow in the proximity of the curvatures, with lower intensity and greater oscillations of the shear stress of the wall. On the other hand, decreasing the force of the linear vector toward the aneurysmal sac would reduce the size of the aneurysms and the risk of rupture. Still a greater swirling flow would lead to greater initial endothelial lesion for the aneurysmal formations. Thus, more obtuse anterior angles, with less laminar flow deceleration and less generation of turbulent flow in the vicinity of the carotid siphon, were statistically associated with larger aneurysms, greater risk of rupture and a higher incidence of aneurysm after the carotid siphon; whereas, more acute anterior angles, with greater deceleration of the laminar flow and greater generation of swirling flow in the siphon, were shown to be associated to smaller aneurysms, lower risk of rupture, and a higher incidence of aneurysm in the carotid siphon [49].

High-velocity laminar flow due to a nontortuous carotid siphon would lead to hemodynamic consequences for the other curvatures and bifurcations of the cranial circulation after the carotid siphon, explaining the higher incidence of postsiphon aneurysms and a higher risk of rupture at these sites in patients with higher angles. Stratified analysis of the subgroups by location revealed that aneurysms located in the anterior communicating artery in patients with anterior angle greater than 15.40° presented an 84% greater chance of rupture (p = 0.049), suggesting that the hemodynamic effects resulting from the anatomy of the siphon can persist anatomically after the siphon [49].

These studies have contributed to a better understanding of the geometric risk factors, but little is known about the anatomical changes in the carotid siphon and, consequently, the repercussions of the hemodynamic changes that the mechanisms of neurosurgical interventions could entail. Devices, such as intracranial stents and detachable coils, and even clips of aneurysms can modify the morphology of the carotid siphon and the knowledge of these consequences could be used to obtain better therapeutic results. This becomes even more important considering that one-third of intracranial aneurysms are located in the carotid siphon [4, 32].

1.5. Flow diverter stents

The microsurgical access of carotid siphon aneurysms can often be considered of high technical complexity. In this way, endovascular treatment has become popular as a safe and effective alternative [32–34].

In the last 10 years, a new device for the treatment of intracranial aneurysms has been presenting promising results, the intracranial flow diverter stents (FDS). They are cylinders with walls formed by braided metallic wires configuring extremely diminutive fenestrations. When implanted in the wall of the parental artery, the small fenestrations allow the passage of blood to the penetrating branches, avoiding neurological deficits, but blocking the blood flow into the aneurysmal sac, and leading to thrombosis and subsequent progressive reduction of its volume [32, 33, 41, 43].

It is nowadays believed that such stents, by virtue of their structural conformation of braided wires, would perfectly fit the anatomy of the vessel in which it was implanted [32].

The rupture of intracranial aneurysms continues to be one of the neurosurgical diseases with the highest morbidity and mortality. Despite advances in the knowledge of the causes and evolution of these lesions, the understanding of all etiological mechanisms remains a challenge for modern neurosurgery.

Recently, hemodynamic studies of the interaction between blood flow and the endothelial wall have received increased attention as an important element in the genesis, development, and rupture of cerebral aneurysms [19, 20, 39]. In this context, studies of carotid siphon interactions are especially important because of the anatomical peculiarities of this region and considering that about one-third of all intracranial aneurysms are located there [1, 18, 21].

Studies such as those by Lin et al., Bogunović et al., and Takeuchi et al. showed that vessels with more intense curvatures are related to greater oscillation and decrease of wall shear force [21–23]. The change in direction of blood flow caused by the carotid siphon curvatures would be related to the transformation of the originally linear flow into turbulent flow. This transformation of the flow pattern would decrease and oscillate wall shear stress, which would precipitate the first endothelial changes in the genesis of aneurysm formation or stenoses [24, 25]. Jou et al., using 3D reconstructions of 25 patients with paraclinoid aneurysms, identified that the mean wall shear stress is inversely dependent on the size of the aneurysmal sac and that ruptured aneurysms present a lower mean wall shear stress near the aneurysmal cervix [39]. Zhang et al., also using 3D reconstructions, hemodynamic studies, and the anatomical classification of Zhang, showed that stenotic lesions tend to appear soon after intense carotid siphon curvatures, also evidencing that siphons that present more pronounced curvatures, such as type C, have statistically more stenoses than siphons with softer curvatures [29]. Piccinelli et al. analyzed individually the aneurysm curves of the carotid siphon and showed that ruptured aneurysms are statistically more present in carotid siphon curves of smaller

http://dx.doi.org/10.5772/intechopen.81400

diameter and shorter length, being preferentially located in the external wall of the curvature [27]. Recently, Lauric et al. compared demographic data with 3D angiogram and showed that women have carotid siphons with curvatures greater than men and patients with aneurysms on siphon also present larger curvatures [40]. Lauric et al. evidenced that men generally have carotid siphons with less prominent curvatures than women [40].

In one of the first studies to evaluate geometric and anatomical changes in the carotid siphons after FDS release in the treatment of the aneurysm in this region and its repercussions Waihrich et al. observed that FDS release led to a morphological change in the carotid siphon, characterized by a progressive and statistically significant increase ($p < 0.001$) in the anterior and posterior angles independently of the angiographic result in the O'Kelly-Marotta scale [35, 50]. In addition, the multivariate analysis showed that there is an increase in the frequency of D results progressively in the quartiles of the anterior angle increase, inferring that there is a greater possibility of radiological cure (result D) in larger increases of anterior angle. Despite the progressive increase of the posterior angle after the FDS release, the statistical relation between this increase and the D result by the multivariate analysis was not observed. Probably, this result was due to the smaller magnitude of the posterior angle increase, both after stent implantation (from 3.97° ± 25.06° to 22.05° ± 25.18° vs. 71.98° ± 31.27° to 79, 43° ± 31.80°), and in relation to the result D with non-D (from 8.34° ± 22.21° to 26.78° ± 24.40° vs. 74.67° ± 25.35° to 81.08° ± 33.58°) [36–38, 50].

The FDS technology is based on increasing blood flow resistance in the aneurysm neck, reducing the inflow and outflow of blood into and out of the aneurysmal sac, and stagnating and thrombosing the blood into the aneurysm. However, changes in carotid siphon geometry may be related to a higher probability of cure. It is possible that the increase of the angle and the reduction of the anterior angle curvature lead to a reduction of the hemodynamic stress in the region, that is, the morphological changes would increase the intensity and reduce the oscillation of the wall shear force, contributing to better final results.

The age, in patients under 60 years, also proved to be an independent variable for a greater chance of cure. Lin et al. evidenced in their study that carotid siphons with greater tortuosity present greater technical difficulty for the release of FDS [21]. In fact, patients older than 60 years presented a higher statistical proportion of the more tortuous types of siphons (types S and C, with $p < 0.001$) and statistically lower values of both the anterior angle (6.06° ± 28.49° vs. 18.07° ± 20.26°, $p < 0.001$), and posterior (71.00° ± 37.68° vs. 80.80° ± 27.14°, $p = 0.025$), evidencing the presence of more tortuous siphons in this population [50]. Another important point is that large and giant aneurysms present greater technical difficulty in their treatment and, in addition, often require more time to thrombose completely [6, 42].

2. Cervical internal carotid artery aneurysm

Aneurysms of the extracranial carotid artery (ECAA) are rare, and little is known about its natural history, the etiology is diverse, and most ECAA are asymptomatic and do not grow over time but may progress into a pulsatile mass, cranial nerve compression, or cause a stroke.

Patients with an asymptomatic ECAA have a rate of ischemic stroke in the aneurysm territory of 1.1 per 100 patient years. For patients with an increasing ECAA diameter, intervention may be considered, while in patients with small non-growing asymptomatic ECAA, a conservative approach seems justified [45].

The main cause of the ECAA is atherosclerotic disease, followed by trauma and most aneurysms in 608 on a total of 1239 patients were located in the internal carotid artery, i.e., its cervical extracranial portion in a study by Welleweerd et al. invasive treatment for extracranial carotid artery aneurysms pertains to only 0.6–3.8% of all extracranial carotid interventions. The best medical treatment comprises antithrombotic treatment and regular follow-up. Traditional surgical treatment has been associated with the risk of stroke and cranial nerve damage; whereas, endovascular ECAA repair has only been described in small case series. However, early mortality and number of strokes is low in surgical and endovascular treatment even in the long-term follow-up, supporting the assumption that invasive treatment could prevent stroke [44].

3. Conclusion

The morphological analysis of the anatomy of the carotid siphon revealed a directly proportional relation between the anterior carotid siphon angle and larger aneurysms, a higher risk of rupture, and the location of the aneurysms distal to the carotid siphon.

The use of flow redirecting stents to treat aneurysms in the carotid siphon caused morphological changes characterized by increased anterior and posterior angles. Specifically, the anterior angle increase was associated with better angiographic results, i.e., aneurysmal occlusion at 6 months.

About ECAA treatment, a better knowledge about the natural history and risk of complications of the different treatments is needed in order to get a consensus, the early and long-term outcome of invasive treatment are favorable, despite some cranial nerve damage be possible after surgery.

Author details

Eduardo Waihrich[1*], Bruno Parente[1], Paulo Gonçalves[2], Fabio Fernandes[1], Carlos Ontiveros[1], Camila Ribeiro[3] and Elias Rabahi[2]

*Address all correspondence to: eduwaihrich@gmail.com

1 Sirio-Libanes Hospital, Brasilia, Brazil

2 Base Hospital, Brasilia, Brazil

3 Brasilia University Center, Brasilia, Brazil

References

[1] Caranci F, Briganti F, Cirillo L, Leonardi M, Muto M. Epidemiology and genetics of intracranial aneurysms. European Journal of Radiology. 2013;**82**:1598-1605

[2] Krex D, Schackert HK, Schackert G. Genesis of cerebral aneurysms-an update. Acta Neurochirurgica. 2001;**143**:429-448

[3] Graf CJ, Nibbelink DW. Cooperative study of intracranial aneurysms and subarachnoid hemorrhage: Report on a randomized treatment study, 3: Intracranial surgery. Stroke. 1974;**5**:557-601

[4] King JT Jr. Epidemiology of aneurysmal subarachnoid hemorrhage. Neuroimaging Clinics of North America. 1997;**7**:659-668

[5] Linn FHH, Rinkel GJE, Algra A, van Gijn J. Incidence of subarachnoid hemorrhage: Role of region, year, and rate of computed tomography: A meta-analysis. Stroke. 1996;**27**:625-629

[6] Choi IS, David C. Giant intracranial aneurysms: Development, clinical presentation and treatment. European Journal of Radiology. 2003;**46**:178-194

[7] Schubiger O, Valavanis A, Wichmann W. Growth-mechanism of giant intracranial aneurysms; demonstration by CT and MR imaging. Neuroradiology. 1987;**29**:266-271

[8] Wiebers DO, Whisnant JP, Huston J 3rd, Meissner I, et al. Unruptured intracranial aneurysms: Natural history, clinical outcome, and risks of surgical and endovascular treatment. Lancet. 2003;**362**:103-110

[9] Ronkainen A, Miettinen H, Karkola K, Papinaho S, Vanninen R, Puranen M, et al. Risk of harboring an unruptured intracranial aneurysm. Stroke. 1998;**29**:359-362

[10] Bonneville F, Sourour N, Biondi A. Intracranial aneurysms: An overview. Neuroimaging Clinics of North America. 2006;**16**:371-382

[11] Kyriacou SK, Humphrey JD. Influence of size, shape and properties on the mechanics of axisymmetric saccular aneurysms. Journal of Biomechanics. 1996;**29**:1015-1022

[12] Inoue T, Rhoton AL Jr, Theele D, Barry ME. Surgical approaches to the cavernous sinus: A microsurgical study. Neurosurgery. 1990;**26**:903-932

[13] Parkinson D. A surgical approach to the cavernous portion of the carotid artery anatomical studies and case report. Journal of Neurosurgery. 1965;**23**:474-483

[14] Isolan G, de Oliveira E, Mattos JP. Microsurgical anatomy of the arterial compartment of the cavernous sinus: Analysis of 24 cavernous sinus. Arquivos de Neuro-Psiquiatria. 2005;**63**:259-264

[15] Krayenbuehl H, Yasargil M, Huber P. Cerebral Angiography. 2nd ed. Thieme; 1982

[16] Zhong SZ, Han YJ, Yen WC. Microsurgical Anatomy. MTP Press; 1985

[17] Lang J, Reiter U. Course of the cranial nerves in the lateral wall of the cavernous sinus. Neurochirurgia. 1984;**27**:93-97

[18] Griessenauer CJ, Yalcin B, Matusz P, Loukas M, Kulwin CG, Tubbs RS, et al. Analysis of the tortuosity of the internal carotid artery in the cavernous sinus. Child's Nervous System. 2015;**31**:941-944

[19] Thomas JB, Antiga L, Che SL, Milner JS, Steinman DAH, Spence JD, et al. Variation in the carotid bifurcation geometry of young versus older adults: Implications for geometric risk of atherosclerosis. Stroke. 2005;**36**:2450-2456

[20] Brisman JL, Song JK, Newell DW. Cerebral aneurysms. The New England Journal of Medicine. 2006;**355**:928-939

[21] Lin LM, Colby GP, Jiang B, Uwandu C, Huang J, Tamargo RJ, et al. Classification of cavernous internal carotid artery tortuosity: A predictor of procedural complexity in pipeline embolization. Journal of NeuroInterventional Surgery. 2015;**7**:628-633

[22] Bogunović H, Pozo JM, Cárdenes R, Villa-Uriol MC, Blanc R, Piotin M, et al. Automated landmarking and geometric characterization of the carotid siphon. Medical Image Analysis. 2012;**16**:889-903

[23] Takeuchi S, Karino T. Flow patterns and distributions of fluid velocity and wall shear stress in the human internal carotid and middle cerebral arteries. World Neurosurgery. 2010;**73**:174-185

[24] Sforza DM, Putman CM, Cebral JR. Hemodynamics of cerebral aneurysms. Annual Review of Fluid Mechanics. 2009;**41**:91-107

[25] Malek AM, Apler SL, Izumo S. Hemodynamic shear stress and its role in atherosclerosis. Journal of the American Medical Association. 1999;**282**:2035-2042

[26] Naruse T, Tanishita K. Large curvature effect on pulsatile entrance flow in a curved tube: model experiment simulating blood flow in an aortic arch. Journal of Biomechanical Engineering. 1996;**118**:180-186

[27] Piccinelli M, Bacigaluppi S, Boccardi E, Ene-Iordache B, Remuzzi A, Veneziani A, et al. Geometry of the ICA and recurrent patterns in location, orientation and rupture status of lateral aneurysms: An image-based computational study. Neurosurgery. 2011; **68**:1270-1285

[28] Kim DW, Kang SD. Association between internal carotid artery morphometry and posterior communicating artery aneurysm. Yonsei Medical Journal. 2007;**48**:634-638

[29] Zhang C, Pu F, Li S, Xie S, Fan Y, Li D. Geometric classification of the carotid siphon: Association between geometry and stenoses. Surgical and Radiologic Anatomy. 2013; **35**:385-394

[30] Silva Neto ÂR, Câmara RL, Valença MM. Carotid siphon geometry and variants of the circle of Willis in the origin of carotid aneurysms. Arquivos de Neuro-Psiquiatria. 2012;**70**:917-921

[31] Sangalli LM, Secchi P, Vantini S, Veneziani A. A case study in exploratory functional data analysis: Geometrical features of the internal carotid artery. Journal of the American Statistical Association. 2009;**104**:37-48

[32] Leonardi M, Dall'olio M, Princiotta C, Simonetti L. Treatment of carotid siphon aneurysms with a microcell stent. A case report. Interventional Neuroradiology. 2008;**14**:429-434

[33] Szikora I, Berentei Z, Kulcsar Z, Marosfoi M, Vajda ZS, Lee W, et al. Treatment of intracranial aneurysms by functional reconstruction of the parent artery: The Budapest experience with the pipeline embolization device. AJNR. American Journal of Neuroradiology. 2010;**31**:1139-1147

[34] Moret J, Cognard C, Weill A, Castaings L, Rey A. The "remodelling technique" in the treatment of wide neck intracranial aneurysms. AJNR. American Journal of Neuroradiology. 1997;**3**:21-35

[35] O'kelly CJ, Krings T, Fiorella D, Marotta TR. A novel grading scale for the angiographic assessment of intracranial aneurysms treated using flow diverting stents. Interventional Neuroradiology. 2010;**16**:133-137

[36] Hosmer DW, Lemeshow S. Applied Logistic Regression. 2nd ed. New York: Wiley; 2000. pp. 260-273. Chapter 8

[37] Allison PD. Logistic Regression Using SAS—Theory and Application. North Caroline: SAS Institute; 1999. pp. 48-51. Chapter 3

[38] Barros AJ, Hirakata VN. Alternatives for logistic regression in crosssectional studies: An empirical comparison of models that directly estimate the prevalence ratio. BMC Medical Research Methodology. 2003;**3**:21

[39] Jou LD, Lee DH, Morsi H, Mawad ME. Wall shear stress on ruptured and unruptured intracranial aneurysms at the internal carotid artery. American Journal of Neuroradiology. 2008;**29**:1761-1767

[40] Lauric A, Safain MG, Hippelheuser J, Malek AM. High curvature of the internal carotid artery is associated with the presence of intracranial aneurysms. Journal of Neuro-Interventional Surgery. 2014;**6**:733-739

[41] Munich SA, Cress MC, Levy EI. Flow diversion for the treatment of intracranial aneurysms: Current state and expanding indications. Neurosurgery. 2015;**62**(Suppl 1):50-55

[42] Becske T, Potts MB, Shapiro M, Kallmes DF, Nelson PK. Pipeline for uncoilable or failed aneurysms: 3-year follow-up results. Journal of Neurosurgery. 2016;**14**:1-8

[43] Zanaty M, Chalouhi N, Starke RM. Flow diversion versus conventional treatment for carotid cavernous aneurysms. Stroke. 2014;**45**(9):2656-2661

[44] Welleweerd JC, den Ruijter HM, Nelissen BG, et al. Management of extracranial carotid artery aneurysm. European Journal of Vascular and Endovascular Surgery. 2015;**50**:141-147

[45] Pourier VE, Welleweerd JC, Kappelle LJ, Rinkel GJ, Ruigrok YM, Worp HB, et al. Experience of a single center in the conservative approach of 20 consecutive cases of asymptomatic extracranial carotid artery aneurysms. European Journal of Neurology. 2018;**25**:1285-1289. DOI: 10.1111/ene.13720

[46] Tada Y, Makino H, Furukawa H, Shimada K, Wada K, Liang EI, et al. Roles of estrogen in the formation of intracranial aneurysms in ovariectomized female mice. Neurosurgery. 2014;**75**(6):690-695

[47] Vlak MH, Algra A, Brandenburg R, Rinkel GJ. Prevalence of unruptured intracranial aneurysms, with emphasis on sex, age, comorbidity, country, and time period: A systematic review and meta-analysis. Lancet Neurology. 2011;**10**(7):626-636

[48] Kubo Y, Koji T, Kashimura H, Otawara Y, Ogawa A, Ogasawara K. Female sex as a risk factor for the growth of asymptomatic unruptured cerebral saccular aneurysms in elderly patients. Journal of Neurosurgery. 2014;**121**(3):599-604

[49] Waihrich E, Clavel P, Mendes GAC, Iosif C, Moraes Kessler I, Mounayer C. Influence of carotid siphon anatomy on brain aneurysm presentation. American Journal of Neuroradiology. 2017;**38**:1771-1775

[50] Waihrich E, Clavel P, Mendes G, Iosif C, Kessler IM, Mounayer C. Influence of anatomic changes on the outcomes of carotid siphon aneurysms after deployment of flow-diverter stents. Neurosurgery. 2018;**83**:1226-1233